Confronting an Ill Society

David Widgery, general practice, idealism and the chase for change

Patrick Hutt

with

Iona Heath and Roger Neighbour

**Foreword by
Richard Smith**

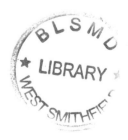

RADCLIFFE PUBLISHING
Oxford • San Francisco

Radcliffe Publishing Ltd
18 Marcham Road
Abingdon
Oxon OX14 1AA
United Kingdom

www.radcliffe-oxford.com
Electronic catalogue and worldwide online ordering facility.

British Library Cataloguing in Publication Data

A catalogue record for this book is available from the British Library.

ISBN 1 85775 910 9

Typeset by Action Publishing Technology Limited, Gloucester
Printed and bound by TJ International Ltd, Padstow, Cornwall

Contents

Foreword

David Widgery – a general practitioner from the East End, political activist, radical journalist, and rock and roller who died young – was about as interesting a person as you could hope to meet. I knew him, and reading this intriguing book has allowed me to rekindle our relationship. I'm confident that others who never knew him will be fascinated to meet him for the first time through this book.

The life, visions, thinking, and excesses of Widgery are well described by Patrick Hutt, a doctor who discovered him posthumously when a disillusioned medical student at Cambridge. Hutt quotes Robert Duncan: 'Though detachment must always be the biographer's aim, he can never achieve it; and more often than not he succeeds in revealing nothing but himself.' He compares his discovery of Widgery to that of a student struggling with the classical guitar who discovers Hendrix, and he manages to present lots of interesting material on Widgery.

But as you read a young doctor writing about his doctor hero you have a feeling of looking into multiple mirrors. Hutt both searches for meaning for his own life as a doctor and tries to make sense of his relationship with his father, who was also a doctor who worked in the East End of London and died young. Hutt was writing the book as his father was dying.

We look into books and see ourselves not reflected but refracted. Therein lies the usefulness and pleasure not only of reading them but also of writing them. We join Hutt and Widgery on a journey where we reflect on what it is to be a doctor, how medicine can be combined with other perhaps more glamorous activities like politics, writing, and rock music, and how we can give meaning to our lives.

Widgery became a doctor partly as 'a debt of honour'. In 1953, when he was 6 years old, he contracted polio and spent weeks in a glass bubble. Hutt decided to study medicine, despite resenting the fact that his father was a doctor, because he was inspired by Iona Heath, another London general practitioner. The power to inspire is one of life's greatest gifts, and Heath, whom I can't resist as describing as wise beyond her 50-something years, contributes to the book a conversation with Roger Neighbour, yet another general practitioner with inspirational talents. Both Heath and Neighbour 'value passion and curiosity in doctors'. These four doctors thus present a rich cache of material for those who want to meditate on the nature of doctoring in general and general practice in particular.

For all of them general practice is not just a job, and perhaps that's true for all general practitioners apart from the most exhausted and burnt out. As a general practitioner you are privileged to learn the secrets of peoples' lives and to be with them in moments of extremity – pain, sickness, and death. If you can empathise, watch, listen, and learn you can understand life and death more deeply than most, as Anton Chekhov, doctor turned writer, showed in his plays and short stories.

Being a general practitioner for these doctors is also a matter of values and politics. They identify strongly with the National Health Service, which continues to embody values of social justice, fairness, and community in a world that sets increasing store by individualism and market forces, which if unrestrained will leave the poor adrift. All general practitioners recognise that poverty, unemployment, poor housing, lack of education, discrimination, and stigma are causes of poor health, but most settle for trying to counter these forces through helping individuals.

For Widgery that could never be enough. He joined the International Socialists, part of what is now called the hard left, and harangued crowds in Chapel Market, Islington. Later, he helped form Rock against Racism and was prominent in the Anti-Nazi league.

Confrontation was part of Widgery's style, and this worked well in yet another outlet for his passion – radical journalism. He was expelled from school for publishing a sexually explicit magazine. At university he started a political magazine called *Snap* and argued that the National Union of Students led by Jack Straw (who is now Home Secretary) was 'financed by a group of CIA bureaucratic fascist bastards'. This was the style of the time, and I was reminded that at a similar age to Widgery I founded a magazine called *BUMp*, which unfortunately was full of adolescent, broken hearted poetry rather than political activism.

Later Widgery was at the heart of a great 60s cause celebre which, like many of them, happened in the early 70s, when the editors of the magazine *Oz* were found guilty of 'conspiring to corrupt public morals' by publishing a 'schoolkids' issue' that depicted Rupert the Bear having sex. (Again in the spirit of how reading sparks thoughts and feelings in us all, I reflect that a friend of mine, now the architecture correspondent of a national newspaper, was on the cover of the corrupting issue.) Widgery kept *Oz* alive by becoming editor.

After writing for many publications Widgery came to write a column for the BMJ. What fun, I thought, that such a radical would be writing in a journal 150 years old and famous for its stuffiness? I'm a great believer in multiple voices in a publication. Impose a party line or an ideology on a journal or newspaper and it will sooner or later lose touch with reality.

'World', says Louis MacNeice in his marvellous poem *Snow*, 'is crazier and more of it than we think/ Incorrigibly plural.' Surrounded by science, numbers, and conservatives Widgery wrote insightful and provocative columns that thrilled many and appalled some. He played an important part in energising the journal and was writing at a time when many felt that the right wing government was tearing the heart out of the NHS. His voice of dissent was much needed.

I find it hard to know how well I knew Widgery. We spoke often on the phone and met occasionally. He asked me to go and speak to the Hackney Philosophy and Literary Society, which he and others had resuscitated after what (I think) was a dormancy of a century. In my (utterly distorted) memory we were revolutionaries gathered around a candle, like characters in a Caravaggio picture. Afterwards, in a manner typical of the 'revolutionaries' I knew, we had a jolly evening in the pub. One of my keenest memories is of Widgery showing me the minutes of a century before, which described how the society had broken up after a debate on the role of women in the society.

Widgery had a wild side to him, loving 'sex and danger'. His heroes, Rimbaud, Shelley, Keats, Hendrix, and Rahsaan Roland Kirk, were prone to dying young, and perhaps it's no wonder in retrospect that Widgery died young. The cause of his death wasn't clear (at least to me), but he had illegal drugs in his body.

The last words that Widgery said to me, shortly after I returned from a year at the Stanford Business School, were: 'I hear that you've been captured by managerialism. We'd better meet and talk about it.' We never did, but I wish we had. He would, I suspect, have been appalled by my development as, I'm fairly sure, he would have been appalled by 'new Labour'. The beauty of this book for me is that it has helped me to have that conversation, albeit in various versions and all in my head. I hope that it will be equally useful to other readers in provoking internal and external conversations. I think it will.

Richard Smith
Editor
BMJ
October 2004

About the authors

Patrick Hutt qualified as a doctor in 2004 having studied at Cambridge University and Barts and The Royal London Hospital. He has a Bachelor of Arts in the History and Philosophy of Science. At the time of publication he can be found answering his bleep at Homerton University Hospital as a Pre-Registration House Officer. This is his first publication.

Iona Heath has been a general practitioner in Kentish Town, London since 1975. She has been a nationally elected member of the Council of the Royal College of General Practitioners since 1989 and has chaired the college's Ethics Committee and its Health Inequalities Standing Group. In 2004, she was appointed to chair the Ethics Committee of the *British Medical Journal* and as a member of the Human Genetics Commission.

Roger Neighbour was a general practitioner in Abbots Langley, Hertfordshire, from 1974 to 2003. He is the author of *The Inner Consultation* (2e)[1] and *The Inner Apprentice* (2e),[2] as well as of numerous papers, articles and opinion pieces on the philosophy of general practice, medical education and the composer Franz Schubert. He was Convenor of the Panel of MRCGP Examiners from 1997 to 2002, and in 2003 was elected to the Presidency of the Royal College of General Practitioners.

References

[1] Neighbour R (2005) *The Inner Consultation: how to develop an effective and intuitive consulting style* (2e). Radciffe Publishing, Oxford.
[2] Neighbour R (2005) *The Inner Apprentice: an awareness-centred approach to vocational training for general practice* (2e). Radcliffe Publishing, Oxford.

Acknowledgements

This work has been hugely dependent on the good will of the many people who knew David Widgery. Special mention must be given to Juliet Ash, who has been generous and open about a subject terribly close to her heart. Similar appreciation can be extended to the many people who gave up time to discuss their old friend and colleague; they appear throughout the text.

Dr Harmke Kamminga must be thanked for getting this project off the ground. The best ideas are never your own. Dr Ashley King, with her Roger Neighbour chat, provided the stepping stone between academic scribbling and the world of medical publishing. Throughout this project there has been no shortage of encouragement. Successive drafts have been shaped by kind critique. Roger Neighbour and Iona Heath have been indispensable with encouragement and advice amidst the lonely world of the redraft. Gillian Nineham and Paula Moran at Radcliffe Publishing deserve credit for their patience and help. Dr Howard Stoate (MP) for giving up time to be interviewed. Thanks must be given to the following people for also offering their comments on various drafts: Paul Julian, Sotirios Zalidis, Becky Ship (it did help), Richard Barling, David Penton and Michelle Malakouna. And to Richard Smith for kindly agreeing to write the foreword.

My thanks to Syd Shelton for his permission to use the photographs on the cover and on p. 19, to Nigel Fountain for the photograph on p. 63 and to Roland Muldoon for that on p. 34.

I must also thank my father. He gave love generously and is missed terribly. A devout sceptic and committed GP, he was never afraid to suggest alternatives. His gentle encouragement remains strong. My mother must be thanked for her critical eye that has continued to flicker since 'advising' me with my English homework. Michelle Dolphin: a big hug. And to my sister, Joanna, who remains immune to medics and their neuroses. There have also been many friends, family and colleagues whose encouragement with this project has been invaluable.

Thanks to the world of medicine must be extended. Both to the experiences and the conversations it produces. Even if it provokes occasional dislike, it remains irresistibly fascinating.

Some characters

Several people appear regularly in the text and need to be introduced. Here are their names and a brief description of their relationship to Widgery. They appear in alphabetical order.

Juliet Ash: Widgery's partner from the late 1970s. Together they formed a loving family, bringing up her son and their daughter. Juliet now lectures at the Royal College of Art.

Kambiz Boomla: an East-End GP who met David Widgery through the International Socialists, and they continued to be active in what it became – the Socialist Workers Party. They worked together on the campaign to save Bethnal Green Hospital. For the slightly younger Kambiz, Widgery was something of a role model. Boomla became chairman of the GPs' East London Medical Committee and a parliamentary candidate for the Socialist Alliance.

Nigel Fountain: generally acknowledged to be David Widgery's best friend. They met during the 1960s. A journalist, Fountain has written a history of the Underground Press and works for *The Guardian*.

Ruth Gregory: worked closely with Widgery on Rock Against Racism, a campaign that was started during the 1970s. A graphic designer, she was responsible for the catchy layout that defined their fanzine, *Temporary Hoarding*. She also worked for the newspaper *Socialist Worker*. She continues to work in the London Borough of Hackney.

Iona Heath: did not know David Widgery personally, but knew of and admired his work. Iona is a leading member of the Royal College of General Practitioners, and has written widely about the role of the GP. Her lectures have reduced people to tears. After feeling let down by New Labour's policies she renounced her party membership shortly after they came to power in 1997.

Roland Muldoon: a member of the radical theatre group CAST (Cartoon Archetypical Slogan Theatre), who looked up to Widgery because they shared an interest in cultural socialist politics. They would meet to debate the issue, usually with the aid of much red wine. Later, when Muldoon took over the Hackney Empire, David Widgery sat on the board of directors. Muldoon and the Hackney Empire continue.

Anna Livingstone: Widgery joined Anna and Tom Kallaway in 1985 at

Gill Street Health Centre, in what later became known as the Limehouse Practice. While Anna has never been a member of the Socialist Workers Party, defining herself as more feminist and libertarian, they shared similar political beliefs. She continues to work in Limehouse and lives with her partner, Kambiz Boomla.

David Phillips: shared a flat with Widgery above Chapel Market, Islington from 1967 to the mid-1970s, when Widgery was a medical student. With Nigel Fountain they composed a political trio which spent a great deal of time in the pub. Phillips is now a lecturer in sociology at the London Metropolitan University.

Michael Rosen: collaborated with Widgery in the 1990s to compose their anthology of dissenting verse, the *Chatto Book of Dissent*. They knew of each other as students but became friends later as Hackney residents. A writer, poet and broadcaster, Michael can be heard regularly on Radio Four. Those with longer memories may remember him on television, playing the role of Doctor Smarty Pants and washing his hair with custard.

Sheila Rowbotham: had a significant relationship with Widgery during the early 1970s. A leading figure in the women's movement (she helped set up the first Ruskin Conference), her ideas are believed to have greatly influenced Widgery. Now a critically acclaimed feminist historian, she lectures at Manchester University and has published many books.

Trevor Turner: knew Widgery from the early 1980s until the time of his death. Now Consultant Psychiatrist and Clinical Director at the Homerton Hospital in Hackney, he and Widgery shared a common belief in a health service for all, free at the point of delivery, but differed over other issues like nuclear weapons. (Turner believes them to be a good way of maintaining the peace, while Widgery wanted them scrapped.) Together they would have long discussions about health politics, typically over a bottle of wine.

Introduction

David Widgery was a socialist GP who worked in the East End of London. As well as being a doctor, he was a father, writer, journalist and activist. For him medicine was as much about the social causes of illness as it was the biological. He believed that if wealth was more evenly distributed, society and its members would be healthier. Widgery defined himself by fighting inequality wherever he could. Working in and fighting for the NHS symbolised his wider view of the world.

The story of David Widgery stands alone. His life was an adventure which could, with a little artistic licence, read like *Treasure Island*. He overcame polio, which left him with a limp, to become not a pirate but a doctor who set sail in search of social treasure. On his journey he came across many obstacles. When his shipmates were imprisoned, Widgery took control of their radical literary vessel – one that went down in the history of British censorship. One day government officials tried to take his hospital away. Rather than give it up, Widgery made it his stockade. Along the way, as friends will testify, there was singing, laughter and the occasional bottle of rum. In his latter years, just as Jim had done before him, he found time to write down his adventures. What happened to the treasure he dedicated his life to finding? There are many opinions. Some say it never existed. Others believe it remains buried just beneath the surface.

While we must be thankful for the rich trail of material Widgery left behind him, this is not *Treasure Island*. The problem with Robert Louis Stevenson's tale is its remoteness. It is escapism in the most fantastic sense. All you can do is dream of pirates and buried treasure as you nod off to sleep. This, however, is the story of an adventure much closer to home. The characters are familiar: the art of medical practice, demanding patients, the National Health Service, government policies, the pursuit of outside interests, keeping hold of what you believe in and the juggling act of life itself.

Some may find Widgery's story causes them to reflect: 'Ah, Widgery went into medicine because of this .... Now why did I go into medicine?' Or perhaps, 'Ah, this annoyed him about practising medicine .... Is there anything similar that frustrates me?' The intention behind this book is not to raise your blood pressure. This may seem paradoxical as you will be thinking about the world of work, which often equates to stress. This need not be the case. Let the mirror become slightly out of focus. These pages represent an escape, a place where ideas can be exchanged freely, with as much or as little weight as desired.

There is a chance that this book will make people happier than they already are. This bold claim is provoked by simple observation. Many in the world of medicine are tired and overworked. Gravity weighs heavy on the eyelids. No amount of caffeine can change that, not once you have passed that point of elasticity. These small but important things are part of wider, deep-rooted unhappiness. In a profession that promises fulfilment, there is a lot of regret. James Le Fanu, in his book *The Rise and Fall of Modern Medicine*, describes the paradoxes of modern medicine. One of them is the increasing number of disillusioned doctors. 'It might be expected that the success of modern medicine should make it a particularly satisfying career, but recent surveys consistently reveal that increasing numbers, especially of younger doctors, are bored and disillusioned. The London-based Policy Studies Institute has found the proportion of doctors 'with regrets' about their chosen career has increased steadily from 14% of the 1966 cohort to 26% of the 1976 cohort to 44% of the 1981 cohort and to 58% of the 1986 cohort.[1]

Medicine in Britain, and arguably all over the world, rests at perpetual crisis point. The actors and circumstances change but the plot remains the same; there are problems wherever you care to look. 'Operation waiting lists could be slashed if hospitals were efficient.' 'NHS trust 'distorted' waiting lists.' 'News analysis: Asthma in British youngsters found to be worst in world.' 'The equipment is just about East European level. It's embarrassing.' 'Angry nurses want 10% pay rise'.[2]

The world of general practice is not immune, the strain reflected by repetitive headlines. In 1999, Dr Ian Bogle, then Chairman of the BMA Council, reported, 'I've been a GP for 37 years. I still think it's the best job in the world, but if I were starting my career now I would be thinking twice before signing up for the abuse, exploitation and oppressive bureaucracy that seem to have become part of the doctor's job description.' At both ends of the spectrum rats abandon and fail to board what they believe to be a sinking ship. Popular sentiment reflects this. Two-thirds of GPs surveyed in December 2002, stated 'morale was low or very low, and a similar proportion said that morale was worse that it had been five years ago. Nearly half would not recommend general practice to an undergraduate or a junior doctor. More than 80% found their work-related stress excessive and 20% found it unmanageable.'[3]

Widgery is an example of resistance to an ethos where standards are becoming more important than the humans they profess to protect. All too often government decisions do not go down well with doctors. Maybe this is the time we live in. Increasing demand for professional accountability and the prioritisation of the consumer have not helped. Decisions are made top down, rather than bottom up. Cynicism and struggling to keep your head above water have become the norm. The bigger questions have no space. What are you meant to do if you disagree with wider trends in medical practice? Is it possible to communicate anything from the coal-face, something that might influence the muffled sounds of policy makers elsewhere? Widgery suggests that self-help is well within our grasp. He possessed skills, as we shall see later, that are now being considered progressive and necessary if doctors are to tackle the sources of their distress.

Widgery draws our attention towards failings that still plague medicine. Inequalities in health have become a depressing fact of life. Someone born into a poor economic status is more likely to die early than someone who is not. If medicine were truly concerned with the prevention of illness, ignoring this depressing fact would seem negligent. David Widgery could not ignore it and did all he could to try and redress the balance. He believed that individuals could make a difference. This may seem idealistic, but therein we find his appeal.

The President of the Royal College of Psychiatrists expressed his concern at the plight of future doctors in these terms: 'The applicants I meet at medical school are alive with the prospect, as people. Years down the line, when I meet them again in their psychiatry placement, their heads are stuffed so full of lists that they seem to have forgotten how to listen to people. I know lists are important, not least in an exam-obsessed world, but not at the expense of distancing oneself from humanity.'[4]

Today we often appear confused about what, if anything, we believe in. Politics has disenchanted many: fewer and fewer people participate in the democracy which we are so quick to defend. Change is inevitable but is it inevitably bad? Widgery believed it was possible for people to change things for the better. At the centre of Widgery's world would be accessible healthcare for all – hence his belief in the NHS.

This book has been written because for many of the difficult questions, there are no easy answers. What is the role of doctors? Should they embrace or ignore the social causes of ill health? How can we encourage a more collective outlook on the health problems that ultimately affect everyone? Indeed, do we want to? Healthcare for all, free at the point of delivery: outdated or underrated? How can doctors be happier? The scope for reflection is broad but the life Widgery led was wide.

Ultimately this book hopes to instil the idea that health professionals can make a difference to the bigger picture; that they can engage in areas which are not traditionally associated with medical practice; that in so doing, both they and their patients might benefit. What happens outside the consultation has the potential to affect what happens within it. There is no blueprint on how to make a difference. Instead, in the breadth of David Widgery's practice and beliefs, is found a springboard for reflection. Looking at David Widgery's tactics, some might think: 'Ah, maybe I'll give this a go.' Or perhaps, and quite likely, 'What madness! I could never bring myself to do that. And quite frankly I don't see any need.'

Debate and dialogue will always be required. Voices of those who are well established in their medical careers need to be heard. The same is true of those for whom the medical tree's branches remain open. Make no mistake though, this is an interdisciplinary meeting. Patients, politicians, managers, scientists, nurses – they all have a perspective. The problems David Widgery spoke about, while particular to some, should resonate with everyone. They concern society.

The book begins with a conversation between Iona Heath and Roger Neighbour – two established voices in the medical world. We shall overhear them discussing the need for diverse inspiration in medicine. Having eavesdropped on their words, the narrative will begin. Chapter 2, 'Behind every book', serves to expose my genetic and environmental conditioning; to shed light on why someone who is barely a doctor should be telling this tale. After this we shall take a look at David Widgery's life in 'A biographical sketch', highlighting with broad brush strokes the major events of his life. The intention is to provide you with an overview, one that conveys the breadth of his political and literary interests. Watch out: we will learn that for many people his greatest contribution had nothing to do with medicine. In 'Medical reasoning', we shall consider why medicine is at times disheartening, and look at the role of social circumstances and the political-by-definition role of the doctor. This will lead us on to think about Widgery's socialist ideals – what made them compatible with medical practice. Continuing with this theme in 'Changing reality', we shall examine the arenas in which Widgery, the GP, fought for his beliefs. I hope that his methods do not seem too alien and that you might be tempted to try some of them at home.

Special attention will be paid to Widgery's ultimate passion, the written word. In 'Written words prescribed', we'll remind ourselves that he was not the first doctor to write outside the prescription pad; doctors have a predisposition for expression. We will look at the potential of this medium, as employed by Widgery, both as a coping mechanism and as a vehicle for change. Particular focus will be given to his major medical works – two books and a column in a well-known medical journal. We shall look at the impact these had. Time will be taken to look at his literary role models, his burning Romantic drive and his persuasive polemical style.

'Wider than Widgery' represents a brief pause. We shall be reminded that he was not the only political doctor. In fact there are many variations on the theme. Returning to Widgery, we shall look at how his role related to the wider political spectrum. It will be argued that his wide appeal lay in medical normality.

Heroes walk on earth not clouds. In the penultimate section, 'Dissecting Widgery', we shall try and understand how Widgery achieved all that he did. We will look at the kind of person he was and how his wider activities related to medical practice. It will be argued that his life was often a delicately poised juggling act which, although impressive, sometimes resulted in turbulent collisions. We shall try and understand the component parts of the fuel that made him burn so brightly.

There are many strands to David Widgery's life, as will become apparent, that have not been explored in detail. The aim has been to keep the focus on medicine and how this related to his wider activities. The closing section draws the threads of the book together. I will share some closing thoughts about Widgery's relevance to medicine today, and thereby tomorrow.

My own life as much as my politics, tells me that the level of compassion with which a society treats its sick and crippled, its old and its feeble-minded, is the real measure of that society's level of civilisation. It tells me that we need a society centred around good health rather than a health service snuffling after disease like a baffled bloodhound. It tells me not that the NHS has failed, but that it has not been given a real chance. This book will have been worth writing if it convinces more people that the health service is something worth fighting for. And that, in fighting for it, we may glimpse our potential to create a society run on a different and better basis.[5]

David Widgery

Firework displays have the power to illuminate, shock and delight. Our heads are constantly turning to catch the next flare-up. David Widgery was a walking November the Fifth. He would not and could not be tied down to a one-track life. For a generation of London's East-Enders he was 'Doc', the GP at the end of hours in the waiting room or the GP who belted round housing estates of Tower Hamlets. But he was also the spirit that raged at the evidence that the diseases he was diagnosing were really diseases growing out of lousy housing, hazardous work and lack of *money*.[6]

An obituary by Michael Rosen

David never conformed; moderation was not a word he understood in anything. He had a voracious appetite for life and an ability to make leaps that left his enemies – and friends – open mouthed. For many on the Left he became part of the intellectual landscape.[7]

Nigel Fountain

Even among rich nations there are many examples of growing socioeconomic inequalities in health over the past 20 years. Health inequalities in Britain have just been declared the worst ever. The life expectancy gap between professional and unskilled workers is now 9.5 years for men and 6.4 years for women.[8]

A Haines, I Heath and R Smith

For

Jo and Nick

(Mum and Dad)

Chapter 1

A conversation about heroes between Iona Heath and Roger Neighbour

RN Iona, I don't know whether you'd agree that sometimes *how* a story comes to be told is a story in its own right. So I thought people who are going to read Patrick Hutt's account of the life of David Widgery might perhaps like to know why you and I are chipping in our two-penn'orth. I believe you know Patrick and his family personally, but I'm not sure whether you knew Widgery himself.

IH I never knew David Widgery personally, though obviously, working in North London as he did, I knew *of* him. And I know a lot of people who knew him – so I suppose I'm at one degree of separation. I knew Nick Hutt as another inner London GP and as Patrick's father, but I didn't know him well. I wish that I had. Patrick – I've known since he was eleven. He and my son Eric were in the same year in the same comprehensive school in Hackney and they became good friends during the first year, and remain so.

RN My involvement is rather more fortuitous. Early in 2001, I was having dinner at High Table at my old Cambridge college, Kings, as you do ...

IH No, some of us don't!

RN ... and was seated next to Dr Ashley King, the Director of Studies in Medicine. She told me about one of her recent third-year undergraduates who, as a dissertation for his Part II in History and Philosophy of Medicine, had written about Widgery in a way that both she and the Tripos examiners had admired. She spoke with such warmth that I asked to read it, and was hugely impressed. I think both you and I value passion and curiosity in doctors; and, after many years spent trying to inculcate these qualities in vocational trainees, it was humbling to be reminded that they are probably there in medical students right from the start.

Cynic that I am, however, I also found myself asking two questions. What was it about Widgery and his 'social activist' style of general practice that could command the admiration of a pre-clinical medical student at an ancient university? And would that admiration survive his clinical training, which is often accused of stifling the idealism of youth?

IH Knowing more of Patrick's background, I think that it is a little easier for me to understand why he should find inspiration in the life of David Widgery. The comprehensive school in Hackney was magnificent in many ways but it was also quite a tough environment. Its great achievement was a genuine aspiration to equality of opportunity for all. I suspect that Patrick found the transition from this to the undoubtedly privileged atmosphere of Cambridge to be quite difficult and that he resented much of the world he had become a part of. I think that David Widgery would have recognised this resentment.

RN I know something that interests both of us is the role that heroes play in people's professional motivation. So what astonished me when I first read Patrick's manuscript was that someone so early in a medical career had such a focused and personalised sense of a doctor-hero. I wondered how he had come by it in the first place. And I wondered what would happen to it en route, because when he wrote the first draft Patrick was still a pre-clinical student. I had a sinking feeling that idealism like his is the sort of thing that gets beaten out of you, or trained out of you, over the next three years at medical school.

IH Yes, unless you find other role models.

RN It's quite hard to preserve that particular form of idealism – and yet one wishes people could.

IH Speaking personally, I've found heroes immensely useful, mostly for how they write. Certainly for me with David Widgery it's been his writing – which is, of course, the only way Patrick had of relating to him, through his writing. That, and a certain amount of London East-End mythology. But it's how people think about what we're doing that, for me, makes them heroes.

RN Who have been your own heroes?

IH My personal enduring hero was John Berger. Then there's been Carl Edvard Rudebeck in Sweden. I heard Rudebeck speak at a conference in Denmark in 1994. He has this fantastic thesis about 'bodily empathy' – how doctors combine their own subjective experience of the body with their objective scientific knowledge of it. This interface is where we work – and actually we have it within us. All the time we're listening to patients, we project that into our subjective impression of our body.

RN In 1994 you would have been in practice for some time; a lot of your professional ideas and values would have established by then.

IH Exactly – and then I suddenly heard Rudebeck speaking about general practice in a way I'd never heard before. It was fantastic. He wasn't necessarily saying anything new – indeed, he was only putting into words things I already knew – but he put them across in a way that made it clear to me that I understood and believed them. That's what I like about your own writing.

RN And I about yours! But enough mutual admiration; what about your earlier hero?

IH John Berger. I was astounded when I recently came across my copy of his book *A Fortunate Man*[9] to see that I'd first read it when I was 19. I don't know how, at that age, I understood any of it. At any rate, when I re-read it 20 years later it came as a complete revelation. But I must have got *something* out of it at 19, because I've always known I wanted to do general practice and I've always had a strong dislike of social injustice. So Berger's book must have resonated at some level with my own values. But what about you, and your heroes?

RN The people you've been describing impinged on your career mainly through language, through speech or writing. By contrast, most of the people I think of as my heroes were not medical. I've been struck more by their personality than by their writings. Peter Tomson, my trainer, for example. He had, for me (in much the same way as Widgery has for Patrick), an ability to point out the things that matter. Before that, there were two teachers at school. One was my biology teacher, Willy Wiles, who just personified enthusiasm for his subject. Even if you were a classical historian, he couldn't fail to make you fascinated by biology. And that was a real ability – it's something to do with energy, and humour, and quirkiness. The other was Frank Thomas, who taught classics and conducted the school orchestra – not always terribly well. But he again had this sense of being driven, and what he was driven to was performing music. Generations of school kids were made passionate about music. It was Frank who introduced me to the music of Schubert, who is also, posthumously, one of my heroes. I wrote somewhere, 'Whereas with Mozart at his best we scale the heights and come down again, when Schubert is at his best we can plumb the soul's absolute depths and come up again.' Which I suppose is a bit like what doctors do; we are with our patients when they're plumbing their own depths and we try to help them come up again.

So you and I seem to have been inspired in different ways by our heroes, you more by their writings and I by personal encounters.

IH Yet saying that, I remember one English teacher who we had for just one term. She impressed upon us, 'Whatever you write about, give examples' – an early defence of the anecdote. It's that thing about detail being important, generalisations are hopeless, you have to get down to the nitty-gritty.

RN Do you think we're talking about two different types of heroism? Could there be one kind of hero who makes us aware of what is possible, by articulating thoughts or values which are latent but hadn't hitherto been expressed? And another more practical kind, whose heroism lies in being a living example of how ideals can be practised and made real? Or maybe it's just that the second kind is simply braver than the first.

IH I've come across a quotation to the effect that heroism is about saying 'yes'. We usually define ourselves in relation to things we reject – I *don't* believe this, I *won't* do that. But heroism is more about the things we accept, the things we *will* do, the things we *do* stand for. Yes, here we are: the Polish poet Czeslaw Milosz. In his Nobel Lecture on 8 December 1980, he said, 'I feel we should publicly confess our attachment to certain names because in that way we define our position more forcefully than by pronouncing the names of those to whom we would like to address a violent "No".' It's through acknowledging our heroes that we are able to declare our aspirations and to define our position in the world. My feeling is that the example of David Widgery has helped Patrick to begin to do this. I think one of the things that Patrick gets from Widgery is the legitimacy of feeling angry . . .

RN Yes, I'm sure that's right.

IH . . . and feeling angry *on behalf of other people* is an important thing for a would-be doctor to feel. And yet social anger, if we can call it that, is historically weakened at the moment, compared with, say, the 1930s, which were riven with social anger. Our society has a lot of individual anger, micro-social anger, frustration and aggression, fed by lack of opportunity.

RN But not that loftier kind of 'anger by proxy', on behalf of other people. I wonder why not; certainly in terms of health inequalities we've probably got *more* to be angry about now.

IH The disadvantaged seem to have become much more varied and diverse – and much more fragmented, less socially cohesive.

RN That cohesiveness has been partly replaced by a sense of impotence – and not just among the disadvantaged. I can imagine a lot of Patrick's readers, including doctors, thinking, 'Well yes, there are things I feel strongly about in my neck of the woods, but I can't see myself ever going to Widgery's lengths.' And they – we – would probably justify that inertia by saying there's no point, or there's no need, or we should abide by due democratic process.

IH I think there are several reasons for the inertia. One is that the young feel politically disempowered – not politically apathetic, but disempowered – because the really large manifestations of ordinary people's outrage, like the miner's demonstrations under Mrs Thatcher and the anti-war protests more recently, are ignored and seem to make no difference in high places. Another reason may be that we don't set them particularly good examples of what it is to be a politically aware professional. Advocacy is a form of structural therapeutics. Professionals have a responsibility to speak out if social injustice undermines people's health, yet we often fail to do so.

RN   Confession time. As you know, I've been a College examiner for a long time, and in the MRCGP exam we ask lots of questions about 'the doctor's role'. The candidates all say, and we the examiners encourage them, 'it's to be the patient's advocate'. But we collude – examiners and candidates – in not meaning what Widgery meant by being an advocate; not 'getting in there, hackles-raised advocacy with the gloves off'. Most of the time we mean something pretty lukewarm, like dashing off the occasional letter to the housing department.

IH   The trouble is, the only way we can have an impact on a wider social stage is by using patients' private stories and telling them in public. And that, of course, is fraught with difficulty, not least because asking consent alters the relationship in a difficult way. David Widgery did it frequently, though I don't know how much consent he ever got.

RN   It's in some way parallel to what Patrick is doing with the now-dead David Widgery – telling his story in order to make social points to a fresh generation.

IH   That's all we ever do, isn't it, when you and I write? There aren't that many completely original ideas to be had, so what one is doing is picking things up from other heroes, repackaging them, giving them one's personal 'take' and trying them out on the readership.

RN   I'm sure that's true. And the irony is, if we wrap them up well enough, people think the ideas are ours.

     Another thought I had about heroes is that they are people who have the ability to induce change at a distance. If you have a one-off encounter with a charismatic speaker or a persuasive writer, they may leave you buzzing with energy, which may or may not last. But the examples we've given of our own heroes were able to have lasting effects on us despite being distanced in time or place or even by death. I wish I knew what the secret is of being able to induce improvement remotely in other people.

IH   It's to do with resonance, isn't it? Some poems, or some paintings or pieces of music resonate for you, and some people do too, while others, with the best will in the world, just don't. John Berger says you have to be looking in the same direction. Let's take medical education as an example. Much of it is conventional, well demarcated, everyone knows the traditional ways of doing it. But what is exciting is when you see someone doing the job who has come out of the same sausage machine, but who has drawn inspiration from completely unrelated areas. For example, I really admire Per Fugelli as a teacher. In his lectures he will cite – completely impartially – Doris Day, Goethe, Aristotle, Billy Ocean. He has an immense cultural grasp, which he can call upon to intensify whatever point he's making.

RN I'd like to stay with the issue of education. The other strand that occurred to me when I first read Patrick's text was what a contribution education can and should make to the process of giving students ideals. We all know how poor or insensitive education can crowd *out* idealism, but I don't know whether the converse is possible. Can we structure education to factor idealism *into* medical students' development? I know some courses try, by having sessions on fine arts or literature – but it often seems to be done rather self-consciously ...

IH ... with lists of approved books: 'This literature is good for you.'

RN Exactly. I call it 'the Middlemarch myth' – that reading about Dr Tertius Lydgate will make you into a good doctor.

IH It's a good deal more complicated than that. If you look at a tree, for instance, as a walker, as a forester, a wood merchant, a farmer, a naturalist, an artist – you see different things in the tree. If you look at a human being as a doctor, as a relative, as a friend, an employee, you see different things in the person. And as doctors, particularly as generalist doctors, we want to enrich our view and make it as huge as we can, so we need as many perspectives as we can. David Widgery gives us a new perspective on ourselves, our job, our patients.

RN That's true; but not everybody who comes across Widgery will resonate on the same frequency as him. I guess that to resonate to a particular hero or a particular source of energy, you have in some way to be pre-tuned by your own personal history. And it's possible to go through life pre-tuned and ready to resonate, yet never come across your particular resonator. I suppose the educational lesson is that we mustn't have too many preconceptions about who should be the heroes for our students. Anybody or anything will do, as long as the student responds. So a curriculum that wants to foster idealism should set its objectives (in the jargon) at the 'meta' level – discover your *own* heroes, don't just adopt the traditionally prescribed ones.

IH It would be good if educationists would read Patrick's book, and think about role models and how to get students to identify their own. There tends to be an assumption that a role model should be someone local and prestigious, like your trainer or the consultant on your firm, whereas we're wanting people to cast much more widely.

RN Agreed. I'd hope medical teachers would take home a message something like, 'You can see from this what a powerful thing having a hero can be. Don't necessarily adopt Widgery as one of yours, but reflect upon who your *own* heroes are and help your students to discover theirs.' And, of course, it doesn't just have to be anger that a hero inspires us to. It could be humour, or equanimity, or wonder, or curiosity, or the capacity to weep.

IH On that note, let's get out of the way so that Patrick's text can speak for itself.

Chapter 2

Behind every book

There is no such thing as complete objectivity especially in human relationships and we delude ourselves when we pretend that there is. Though detachment must always be the biographer's aim, he can never achieve it; and more often than not he succeeds in revealing nothing but himself. This being so, perhaps he should in the first place admit to those factors which have probably limited his vision and thus give the reader the chance to make adjustments accordingly.[10]

Ronald Duncan

There are so many voices in this world. Most are merely whispers on the wind, but some voices are heard more clearly than others. The temptation is to suspect that such voices are heard, not simply because they are louder, but because they amplify whispers already present. This was certainly the feeling I had when I discovered David Widgery. Much of what he sought to achieve with his life resonated strongly with me. This is what prompted me to write, believing that his story has the potential to inspire others.

The writing of this book has overlapped greatly with my own life. It was written in its original form roughly halfway through my undergraduate medical training. Up until that point I had felt rather uncertain and uneasy about medicine. From my own experience with medical training, it had been easy to feel committed to a single-track life. The current was strong, pulling me towards land visible years before I arrived. Messages travelled quickly on the ocean breeze. The long hours, poor staff morale, the general doom and gloom; they all lead you to believe that medicine is no paradise. As reality takes over, ideals become distant memories. People will say, 'I used to be idealistic, but you soon realise that's impossible. Are you sure you want to do medicine?' To study and practise medicine can be to become cynical and to forget. Widgery helped me believe that this need not be the case.

My father was a Hackney GP. It was in this London borough that I grew up. For many years I resented the fact that my father was a doctor. People would pose the obvious question, 'So what are you going to be when you grow up?' Astronaut (I first thought), or fireman, or footballer, tennis player, architect, physicist, barrister, haven't a clue. But even before I got a chance to answer, people would interrupt. 'I knew it! You're going to be a doctor ... just like your father.' I would adamantly deny this; in my world, 25% of pupils struggled to achieve five GCSEs, grade A–C.[*]

In truth, I was never especially interested in sciences. It all seemed so boring. Copy out of the textbook and recite. Copy out of the textbook and recite. That was how GCSE science was taught and passed. Like many calculating souls I studied A-level subjects that were not necessarily my favourite. I preferred history and English literature. But I chose sciences after being told, 'The arts are always accessible in later life. They are located in the public libraries. All you need do is pick a book off the shelf. It is much harder to return to the sciences.'[11] My philosophy was about keeping options open. Doing chemistry meant that medicine was not completely ruled out.

Science changed for the better at A-level, which had everything to do with enthusiastic teaching. Through simple thought the universe was bought to life. With harnesses and ropes, students oscillating from ceilings demonstrated simple harmonic motion. Mr Peter Campbell told us we had to be inquisitive, to ask questions like a child. We should be amazed that things fall off tables and crash to the ground (words that were performed with the simultaneous action). Outside reading helped. Primo Levi showed that chemistry could be bonded with humanity, while Richard Feynman articulated what a fascinating thing science could be. 'If you are going to teach people to make observations, you should show them that something wonderful can come from them ... In religion, the moral lessons are taught, but they are not taught once – you inspire again and again, and I think it is necessary to inspire again and again, and to remember the value of science for children, for grown-ups, and everybody else.'[12]

My decision to study medicine was helped by the 1995 Christmas Lecture at the Royal College of General Practitioners, given by Iona Heath. Talking to 17-year-olds at a time of turmoil, she argued that general practice was the best profession in the world. She highlighted that medicine was not straight science. A healthy interest in the arts was equally important. My thought process went something like this: 'Hang on just a second. I thought general practice was meant to be boring. It's what my dad does. I thought medicine was all about A-level chemistry and reading *New Scientist*. No one ever told me that you could hang about in lavish buildings quoting from impressive-sounding books.' This was the fresh perspective I needed. The spark was fanned by work experience. Patients appealed. Promising myself a third year studying something non-medical, I applied to study medicine at Cambridge.

---

[*] These are the minimum set of grades generally required before you can take the exams required if you are to attend university.

Medical school was a comedown. After surfing the wave of success, I was soon struggling to keep my head above water; weighed down by a heavy workload and lack of confidence that seemed entrenched amongst many. Adding to the splashes of distress was a realisation that many of the things you needed to know to complete a medical degree were not that inspiring. People would say, 'This is rather boring but you simply have to know it.' Biochemistry became the bane of my life, followed closely by the contents of carpal tunnel. Such was the volume of work that there was no time to pause and ponder those subjects I found fascinating, like the body's immune system. It was ridiculously competitive; vomiting and beta-blockers were common conversation around exam time.

People skills, with patients hidden far away, were not part of the equation. At the same time politics and wider issues were not discussed. This seemed ironic; every medical school interview had included a question on the NHS. I became somewhat disillusioned. Thankfully salvation was around the corner.

During my third year at Cambridge I chose to study History and Philosophy of Science. Words cannot convey how refreshing this was. Nothing I had taken for granted could escape the enquiring eye of the philosopher and historian of science. Subjects such as the origins of clinical medicine and the nature of causation were debated. Students were encouraged to express their own opinions and come up with new ideas. This was something medical rote learning did not encourage. I encountered voices so sceptical they refused to believe that anything science told them could be true. Within this fascinating world of ideas the origins of this book are found.

I had to write a dissertation. I wanted to write something about medicine, to try and articulate the spectrum of emotions I had experienced during my odyssey. The problem was that there was so much I wanted to write about. I needed a vessel to carry me. Thankfully my supervisor, Harmeke Kamminga, came up with a good idea.

'Have you heard of David Widgery?'

I had to think twice but the name sounded familiar. She pressed on.

'He was a radical doctor from East London. I think he died not too long ago.'

What memories remained flooded my conscience. Wasn't he that local GP who wrote books about the NHS? Yes . . . that was it. I had attended his memorial with my family at a packed Hackney Empire following his death. I must have been 14 at the time. Speakers from various organisations paid tribute. His daughter played the piano and his stepson spoke about him. A juggler, who threw melons to the circle, entertained. So yes, I had certainly heard of David Widgery but remained almost clueless about who he was. Intrigued, I tracked down a copy of his book *Some*

Lives![13] and set about skimming through it in the cold Cambridge University library. In the space of a few paragraphs I was transported from the studious atmosphere of the library to the seemingly remote memories of my childhood. Here is an extract from the chapter *On Yer Bus*, which I read that day.

> The terracotta muse high above the roof of the Hackney Empire waves people to work, abstractedly. Everyone in a sudden, sodden hurry. A crowd masses and mills the bus stop outside the Central Hall. Between the lurches a woman in mauve overcoat and carpet slippers belabouring the world in torrid patois. Each outburst culminates in the repeated cadence of 'Ras Clat Cunt.' Is she psychotic or just drunk? The school-children scared for a moment, part to let her through, reverting at once to their quarrels ... The kids occupy the front of the bus get still more noisy as they approach the impending discipline of school. 'And then he twines him and blasts the next geezer and just touches it in. Safeness' (football). 'So I just blanks him and he starts giving me licks' (psychology). 'He's a fuckin' African, so how am I supposed to understand him?!' (Afro-Caribbean boy).

At this point I laughed out loud, looking around with embarrassment to see if anyone had heard me. Then again, this time for longer, to see if there was anyone I could share my delight with. The portrayal of the reality I had once known was apt. The vocabulary and behaviour were very familiar to me. To explain: 'safeness' signifies approval. 'Blanks' is to ignore. 'Licks' is to hit someone, more than once. Racism, as the extract conveys, is not simply a black-and-white problem.

It was as though, while struggling to learn the classical guitar, I had finally heard Jimi Hendrix. The more I found out the more intrigued I became. For example, I was tremendously reassured by the fact that Widgery had struggled to decide between the arts and the sciences. He had wanted to do both and had ultimately managed to organise his life so that this was possible. At the same time, his passage through medical school had not been one of unadulterated success. He questioned what many took for granted.

I was able to draw parallels between his experience and my own. Rightly or wrongly, I was bothered by the fact that 50% of Cambridge undergraduates were from private schools despite making up only 7% of the general school population. (This is usually explained by the fact that not enough state school students apply and that only the best students are chosen, regardless of where they went to school.) On top of this I was shocked by the lack of ethnic diversity (this can be partially explained by a Hackney upbringing). I took solace in discovering that David Widgery highlighted far more troublesome statistics when he was at medical school during the 1970s. You were more likely to get into medical school if you were male, white and your parents had studied there (fine for me but not for most of my sixth form). I am not suggesting he alone was responsible for the change, simply that some of his views were accepted, over the course of time, to be right.

Later, as I moved into the world of clinical medicine, I kept his story close at hand. Here are two examples where thinking of Widgery helped me cope. In one clinic, after saying goodbye to a charming family, the doctor turned to me and said, 'You really do meet some wonderful people in this profession. It's a shame not all patients are like that, some are really ungrateful. Take all these blacks; they sit around in their council houses, unemployed, complaining all the time. They are so lazy.' On another occasion, we were being taught about chest x-rays. Our mentor decided to let us into a secret. 'What test do you want to do if you see a nipple ring on a male x-ray?' We were all baffled. Smiling shrewdly the teacher said, 'HIV'. Then he revealed the line of thought: nipple ring, homosexual, cough, therefore HIV. I am not suggesting that these incidents are typical of my medical education, but the taste of sour milk lingers however quickly you try and forget.

Widgery also seemed to care about the NHS. He believed that it was important to have a healthcare service that looked after everyone, not simply those who could afford it. While there are many people who believe this, it is often hard to hear them say it. On the other hand, a variation of the following can be quite common, 'It's rubbish. Get out while you can. You really don't want to become a doctor.' The negative prevails, not with a belief that things can get better, but that it will only get worse. Understandably, it is frustrating There are many problems but there are many good things too.

Reading Widgery, I realised that my sentiments were not totally out of place. When it counts, the NHS is more likely to be there than not. David Widgery, as you will soon see, learnt this lesson after great personal tragedies. It inspired him to write, 'In the 1980s, politically dominated by the philosophy of possessive individualism, the NHS still allows a different set of values to flourish.' These words, and the incident that preceeded, have sadly taken on a far more poignant meaning in my life.

In the process of writing this book, I have watched my father die. A malignant melanoma metastasised to his brain. He was 51. There was very little that could be done to save him. Steroids reduced the swelling in the brain. Anti-epileptics were started after he had his first fit. The NHS helped my father die. This may seem paradoxical but it is the truth, from the doctors who spoke to him and the nurses who phoned, to the volunteer at the flower shop who told me he'd collapsed.

There was a reliable structure in place to help him and us, his family, at our most helpless. As my dad tried to make some sense of his predicament he would say, 'That's what the NHS does best, looking after people. I've always believed that.' Science could not save him; but science saves very few people, and ultimately none of us. Medicine can only strive to make the journey of life more bearable. Amongst the tears, my mum would say to me, 'Thank God for the NHS. What would we do without it?'

As I grew older the shame of having a doctor-parent became replaced by a more defensive stance. To go into general practice is still perceived by many as something of a failure. It means being not as good as your hospital colleagues. Ask a student and you will be told, 'GPs are nice people but what a boring job! No one is really ill. You just get to prescribe paracetamol and attempt to convince people that they do not need antibiotics for their sniffles.' What's more, there are people who will suggest that the success of a medical career can be measured by the geographic location in which you practise. East London, with all its crime, violence and poverty, was therefore bottom of the pile. At medical school I struggle to hear anyone saying that they would like to enter general practice. If they do, they reluctantly whisper it.

David Widgery made medicine and general practice seem appealing. Poverty, politics, patients as people – they all mattered. He also helped dispel my remaining adolescent anxiety, which up until that point had been, 'If someone wants to get up and dance that's great, as long as that someone is not my dad.' My father had chosen to work in the East End because he believed it to be something of a noble cause, not simply a second-rate alternative. Everyone fears his or her father might be unfashionable. Believing in the NHS (as he did) is a bit like wearing corduroy trousers, and to be in general practice is to add a tank top with purple circles. I realised my father had been doing a variation of the Widgery. This made me proud, not ashamed.

Chapter 3

A biographical sketch

In his [David Widgery's] dream of dreams for bringing about social change he would have a Tony Cliff or Tony Benn-like figure speaking whilst Miles Davis or Bob Marley played in between speeches. Dave would be smoking a joint whilst the bloke next to him would say, 'Hey doc, I've got a bad leg. You couldn't help me could you?' He was a marriage of so many different things and elements. Very few people that you know would have tried to haul together so many different elements in one life.'[14]

Michael Rosen

David Widgery was born on 27 April 1947. Maidenhead, in Berkshire, provided the setting for Widgery's upbringing. His mother was a primary school teacher and his father Arts Director for ICI. For most children medicine would have been far from their minds, but Widgery was an unfortunate exception.

During the summer of 1953 Widgery contracted polio, he was six years old. No systematic vaccination programme had been introduced to Britain and the consequences of contracting the disease were severe. Widgery was later interviewed by Tony Gould for the book *A Summer Plague: polio and its survivors*. 'At one moment the six-year-old David was lying on a rolled up carpet while his mother hoovered around him, unable to move when she asked him because he felt so tired. The next, he was in one of a row of glass cubicles in hospital saying goodbye to his father.'[15] Sufferers were quarantined from friends and family in a bid to limit spread. 'They were like goldfish bowls ... My mother was allowed to come to the door and read me stories. She read me stories of the stickleback sailor and I hung onto her words. Mothers were only allowed in for half-an-hour a day or something. You cried yourself to sleep, and you'd wake up and then you'd see another little boy crying himself to sleep in the next cubicle. It was awful.'[16] While traumatic, the consequences could have been much worse had someone not intervened.

It [my polio] certainly had a lot to do with my views about the National Health Service and about being a doctor ... It certainly made me very pro-NHS, because I know for an absolute certainty that the treatment I got on the NHS would never have been available on a commercially based system; I would have had to be a millionaire to get the surgery I had. The fact that I got a series of very successful reconstructive operations for nothing on the NHS made me feel there was a debt of honour and I had to pay my dues. Becoming a doctor was partly to do with that, and my political defence of the NHS – which I spend quite a lot of time doing – is partly to do with that.'[17]

Less publicly known was that he also suffered from tuberculosis during his childhood, which left him with an obvious scar on the left side of his neck. It would be nice to imagine Widgery, the fiery youth, determined to become a doctor from the tender age of nine. However, such romantic clichés are best saved for hospital television dramas. He was not thinking of medicine when he decided upon his A-levels, choosing to take English, history and art.[18]

Attending a reputable grammar school, Widgery was expelled for publishing a sexually explicit school magazine, *Rupture*. During this same period he ran away from home, living in a caravan at the bottom of his girlfriend's garden.* Widgery defined himself as an adolescent with a sense of adventure. In his late teens he travelled across America, 'in the throes of the Civil Rights struggle', as described in one of his obituaries. By the end he had 'met some of the first anti-Vietnam activists, fallen in with the Students for a Democratic Society, listened to Roland Kirk [the jazz musician] – and heard him racially harassed – and visited Cuba.'[7]

There was a charming naivety in Widgery's understanding of the political relationship between the USA and Cuba. On the beaches of Miami he went around asking people where he could buy a ticket to fly to Cuba. Such escapades were to become symbolic of the maverick, and often comical, life David Widgery embraced.

It was only after completing school, whilst working as a hospital porter, that Widgery became seriously interested in medicine. This experience rekindled his interest in the sciences. It also allowed him to view the personal interactions that kept the NHS functioning on a daily basis. Juliet Ash, his partner from the late 1970s, believed that there was a political element to his decision. Surprisingly, he never referred to this period in similar fashion to his childhood; the story of an inspired nine-year-old arguably makes better reading. Part of Widgery wanted to become an orthopaedic surgeon, to repay his debt that he felt he owed the NHS. The necessary A-levels were obtained at evening classes whilst continuing to work at the hospital.

---

* This incident is said to have lasted only a few days. It is interesting that her father fought against Franco in the Spanish Civil War.[19]

Applying to study medicine is one thing but to be successful in your application is another. Relatively speaking, the odds were stacked against him. His academic track record was less than sparkling. He had been expelled prior to taking his arts A-levels, and the subsequent grades he obtained in science were not brilliant. These were the factors over which Widgery had control, but at the time of his application it was not purely objective criteria that determined success. The image of the medical school population consisting of doctors' sons from public school was far truer in 1965 than it is today.

There was no one medical in my family: my mother was a primary school teacher, my father had no qualifications at all. I wouldn't have ever dreamt of getting into medicine, nor would I have managed to get in, if I hadn't had this very close experience of the health service as a patient.[17]

How exactly Widgery got accepted to study medicine remains unclear. Juliet Ash got the impression that the Royal Free Medical School accepted one 'risk factor' every year, i.e. a student who did not fulfil the traditional academic requirements. Be that as it may: in 1965 David Widgery entered medical school.

Changing times

The 1960s and early 1970s were a time of social and political upheaval. While it was cool to listen to Hendrix and smoke dope, a political conscience was the ultimate accessory. Many sincerely believed that the world would be shaped and changed on the basis of their actions. Student politics were fuelled by an energy and self-belief difficult to imagine for those who were not part of that generation. There was more to university than obtaining a degree to increase your employability.

In 1965 Widgery came to London. Not long afterwards his two non-medical friends, David Phillips and Nigel Fountain, joined him.* They would while away afternoons in pubs, reading socialist quotes, trying to guess who had said what and when.[20] 'Did Marx or Engels say this?' Their relationship was one centred around beer, politics and laughter. Phillips, now a lecturer in sociology at the London Metropolitan University, reflected on the period:

---

* They had originally met at a student meeting in York.

It is difficult to rekindle the mixture; the music, the politics, the look; long hair, black PVC mac. Widgery had one. And a pair of jeans with so many patches on you wondered where the jeans were. It was terribly exciting and real. It was a reaction to our parents' generation, which now I feel rotten about in a way ... I don't think we appreciated all that they had been through. There was this great crumbling of fixed positions and boundaries, of what was possible. It was a tremendous time of hope in all kinds of ways. Hope for one's self, hope for the future, hope for a better world ... Some of it seemed achievable.

1968 became a symbol for a whole generation that emerged from this period. Ten years later Tariq Ali, a prominent political figure on the Left, wrote 'Revolutionary socialism was reborn in 1968. Its inspiration came from the battlefields of Vietnam and the Sierra Maestra in Cuba, from the barricades of May–June 1968 in France and from the courageous Czechs who confronted Soviet tanks not with grenades, but with political argument.'[21]

A lot was happening politically. Domestic Britain was seen as a microcosm for the world. Students occupied buildings and demonstrated their support for causes a long way from home. The possibility of a global socialist alternative was a reality for many. It was a busy time for the trio who had joined the International Socialists (IS), a small independent left-wing party. 'There was a time,' reflected Phillips, 'when I could look at my diary and know exactly what I was doing for IS every day for a month ahead.' Widgery described walking around London with a transistor radio pressed to his ear, events were moving that fast.[22] Student groups from abroad would come and visit, exchanging ideas on political activism. On one occasion German Students for a Democratic Society came to discuss tactics for dealing with the police. Previously the tactics of IS had been no more than an enthusiastic and rather English gesture of 'link arms, comrades'. Phillips remembers his astonishment at the visiting students, who 'were something else! With proper military formation and tactics.'[19]

London was an exciting place to be, especially for the boy who had grown up in Maidenhead dreaming of revolution. Politics was only part of the equation. There was a 'happening' social scene that Widgery could not resist. As best friend Nigel Fountain explained, 'Coming to London was excitement. Political excitement, getting drunk, beautiful women, glamour and so on ... David was very attracted to that. He was simultaneously attracted to it and appalled by it. The ideal combination was to go along to a party and denounce everyone.'[20]

Widgery was also rather popular with women, conducting a string of relationships during his life. Something in his personality was obviously responsible. David Phillips attempted to put his finger on it. 'He was a very magnetic person. You could just sense it. He was that blend of sex and danger. He was attractive. He looked a bit like David Bailey; straight black hair and Adriatic eyes. He would have been six-foot four had his legs not been pinned after polio. This made him about five-foot eight. He had a big torso above short legs. He certainly had this sense of power that he radiated. They wanted to tame him, to get him in their web.' Fountain adds the cautionary note, 'They would usually end up chasing him round the room with a rolling pin.'

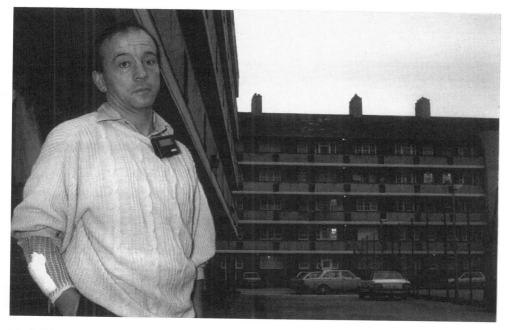

Dr Widgery poses for a photo in his book *Some Lives!* The caption for which read, 'On Sunday evening call out, St Vincent's Estate, Limehouse ... recently mugged.'

Party politics

Having joined IS, all three friends attended regular meetings held above a pub in Chapel Market, Islington. Numbers were small and the atmosphere relaxed. 'It was more anarchic, more libertarian,' Nigel Fountain recalled.[20] Influential people like Tony Cliff, Chris Harman and CLR James would regularly attend. When the group became too big, it subdivided to become the Angel IS branch. Phillips became the secretary whilst Widgery became 'the charismatic leader figure'.[19]

IS was a political party based around local activism. As Fountain explained, 'We were taught that because we were International Socialists we had to go out and organise at a grass-roots level. This involved selling *Socialist Worker* [the official paper of IS] and organising on the [local housing] Estate. This would often come down to selling *Socialist Worker* on the Estate.'[19]

IS was a valuable experience for Widgery. It gave him a structure to harness his more radical inclinations. Rather than being angry with the world, it instilled the belief that it was possible to do something constructive to change it. Fountain describes how 'one side of David was the anarchic and exploding. Another side was very determined and organised. One of the virtues of IS was that it provided him with a body of theory. It provided him with a built-in commitment.'[23]

On Saturdays they would drag a heavy fold-up platform, constructed from wood by Widgery and Phillips, from one end of the market to the other. The afternoon would be spent standing on it, addressing shoppers at the busy Chapel Market. Verbal confrontations became inevitable. There was always a measure of public hostility. Speakers would be forced to listen to arguments about 'blacks taking all the jobs' and how students like Widgery should 'stop sponging off the state and get a job'. It was an eye-opening experience for the trio, all of whom had attended grammar schools outside London. Fountain explained, 'I was forced to go and stand on a platform at the end of Chapel Market and harangue the crowds. David and I were there at the time of Vietnam. The point was that we encountered a milieu we had never encountered. You started having political arguments with other people.' Through contact with 'a small cadre of interesting working-class intellectuals' who attended the IS meetings, 'a lot of cramped lower-middle-class attitudes' were broken down. It was a skill that Widgery carried with him for the rest of his life. He was never afraid to address people who did not agree, to engage those who others might ignore.

At the same time, there was a prevailing sense that genuine workers, the people most valued by IS, were a rarity. When one did turn up to a meeting members would be fascinated to hear their story, eager for a genuine account of what it was like to be on the shop floor. Phillips felt these new recruits were more interested in the end of the meeting, when they could drink the beer and 'run off with the girls'.[19] He also questioned the degree of Socialist triumph on the local housing estates. The man who had been encouraged to set up a tenants' group said, 'It's worked very well actually. We got the kids to stop putting dogs in the spin dryers!'[20]

Radical writing

Widgery was working hard to establish his name, not as a conscientious medical student, but as a radical writer. One of his first efforts was producing a magazine called *Snap*. Providing an alternative view of student politics, Widgery criticised the then President of the National Union of Students. Nigel Fountain humorously recalls, '*Snap* was waging war on Jack Straw [president of the NUS 1969–71, representing the Radical Student Alliance]. Widgery was so right about Jack Straw. Widgery was anti-leadership of the NUS. He argued that the NUS was financed by a group of CIA bureaucratic fascist bastards, all of which was broadly speaking true. More specifically, Fountain explains that Widgery was critical of such broad, inclusive and compromising left-wing politics.

Widgery was not the only dissenting writer. Many people were publishing their own work in a movement that became known as the Underground Press. Pamphlets, newspapers and magazines were produced to counterbalance the mainstream. One of the most famous magazines in this genre was a psychedelic publication called *Oz*. Many of today's social commentators like Germaine Greer were found within its pages. David Widgery became *Oz*'s political writer and was noted for his inability to spell 'Guevara' correctly.

In 1971 *Oz* came to the forefront of national debate. An issue compiled by teenagers, which was to become known as the *Schoolkids' Issue*, provoked a huge reaction. Its editors, Jim Anderson, Richard Neville and Felix Dennis, were accused of 'conspiring to corrupt public morals and possessing, publishing and spreading obscenity'.[24] Central to the outrage was that one of Britain's favourite childhood characters, Rupert the Bear, was depicted having sex. The trial, during which the editors were imprisoned, was a key moment in the history of British censorship. Widgery stepped in as editor to keep *Oz* alive.

Looking back from a distance, we might assume that all people who read *Oz* were radical. But simply buying *The Guardian* does not make you left wing, as Widgery was quick to remind his readers. In particular he was scathing about hippies. As Phillips explained, 'Once you were into [socialist] politics you were critical of the hippies and 'lifestyle' politics. You thought it was all a bit indulgent, not really focusing on the world which needed changing.' These sentiments come across strongly in the following extract from one of Widgery's articles in *Oz*:

> The more the underground loons on about the revolution, the more obvious it becomes that pot (marijuana) serves roughly the same role that gin did in the 1920s, to enable the enlightened to sit about talking

about their enlightenment. The club called 'Revolution' where youthful members of the ruling class whinny under the portraits of Mao and Che is typical. The hippies in Britain are about as much threat to the state as people who put foreign coins in gas meters.[25]

The surreal

Through his writing and his politics Widgery made links. Seemingly unconnected interests would become part of his socialist vision. In *Oz* Widgery did his best to politicise the psychedelic movement, to introduce socialism and argue against the war in Vietnam. (Looking back on the period he wrote, 'It was Vietnam, almost Vietnam-as-metaphor, that impelled psychiatrists to discuss imperialism and hippies to encounter Marxism.'[26]) This skill, of joining outlying dots, was applied to his public speaking. Ruth Gregory, a graphic designer who worked closely with him on a later project, appreciated this. 'You'd never fall asleep when he was talking. He was very funny, lively. Just leapt around all over the place, so he'd keep your mind going. Always, even if it was about the past, he was always referring it to the present. Making a straight connection.'[27]

Such attributes were in stark contrast to what most had come to expect when attending political meetings. Phillips explained that Marxist meetings normally consisted of 'reports of strikes, or you'd get some canon of the Russian Bolshevik Party. Widgery mingled Marxist analysis with stuff about contemporary rock music and what was going on in the newspapers, which was quite unusual – the way he could make these connections.' This unique style was responsible for increasing the party's appeal. 'People who were coming into IS were not from families who'd been on the left for donkey's years. People who came fresh found people like Widgery very exciting. He provided alternative socialism that joined up things we were into. He was very against the puritanical, what you might call the old left; the dreary side of the left. And boy, can it be dreary.'

The traditional political parties of the left had their problems. As Roland Muldoon, member of the radical theatre company Cartoon Archetypical Slogan Theatre (CAST), explained, 'The Communist Party had to defend Russia. Labour had to defend being pro-United States. So they were completely flawed.' Nevertheless most socialists appreciated the need for a party. 'You wanted some kind of orthodoxy, a machine, because you were political activists. But the trouble with it was that it went Stalinoid, in itself it became "The Party". The Party became illiberal.' Muldoon was not a member of any political party, but IS was the party with which he identified most. This was largely due to the presence of David Widgery.

Widgery loved 'beat poetry, radical literature and jazz'.[19] He believed that culture shaped people's views of the world. Culture was political. It could be used for good and for bad. CAST shared a similar view and was inspired by Gramsci, the founder of the Italian Communist Party. Muldoon explains how Gramsci's 'idea of building a party was tied up with culture. The reason why the Italian Communist Party kept on so long was because you had this whole big cultural thing, the fairs and the festivals, this involvement of people.'[28] That Widgery shared a similar analysis meant he was revered. But it was not only that. He was a dissenting voice within IS, speaking out about things which would otherwise have remained unsaid. Although IS was 'progressive' it was also conservative in many ways. Fountain and Phillips at times despaired of the leadership. 'IS ignored the women's groups that we were into. It regarded them with great suspicion, as a diversion to the working classes. As for Gay Liberation, they regarded it as absolutely appalling, something that would put off workers from joining the organisation. Even a thing like racism was regarded as secondary to class-based politics.'[19]

David Widgery would have none of it, sticking his neck out about sexism, homophobia and racism. 'A male worker who sneers at queers, just like one who talks of niggers and slags, is finally only sneering at himself and at his class,' he said. This breakaway stance meant he softened people's despair with left-wing politics. Friends credit his relationship with the historian Sheila Rowbotham for successfully fulfilling this role.

Fountain believed Widgery developed from this a 'sense of history and learning. A way of looking; he already had it but it emphasised his role of the dissident even within the IS.' It also exposed him to feminist arguments which he employed in other arenas. Widgery pointed out to his readers that the 1960s' sexual liberation seemed to benefit one sex preferentially. 'Women are doubly enslaved, both as people under capitalism and women by men. The hippie chick has always been one of the most unfree of women; assigned to be ethereal and knowing about Tarot and the moon's phases but busy at cooking, answering the phone and rolling her master's joints.'[29] This maverick side, often at odds with the leadership of IS, was tolerated because the party could ill afford to lose him. It led Bob Light, a prominent member of the party, to describe him as 'a radical humanist intellectual on permanent loan to revolutionary socialism'.[30]

Disillusioned student

If you did not already know it, you might be surprised to learn that David Widgery was training to become a doctor. One of his then flatmates was certainly bemused. 'He was a medical student, but you didn't get any sense that he spent time on it. He certainly wasn't a model student. I mean he had the books. I got the impression that he was focused in the other way, politics and writing. I've never understood the medical training system. But we were young, you know, we had a world to change.'

An obituary published in the *BMJ* described Widgery as 'not the most assiduous medical student'. Medical school for someone like Widgery could not have been an easy experience. The culture predominating in a teaching hospital would have seemed many miles from his political activities and dreams. As Fountain recalled, 'One of the features about his time at medical school was that he was surrounded by a bunch of right-wing medical students. That was one of the reasons Widgery was so happy to see me and Phillips arrive because it meant he didn't have to spend all his time talking to a bunch of people telling him Ian Smith* in Rhodesia was a really good thing.'

Nigel Fountain believed that Widgery 'got out of the frustration by not being there'. He certainly had no qualms about skipping lectures to participate in the 1969 student occupation of the London School of Economics. In 1970 he stopped going in completely.[31] Medicine had obviously become a peripheral priority. It came as no surprise to anyone when Widgery failed his finals, though he retook them successfully in 1972.

Despite his poor attendance and exam results, Widgery was not to be kept silent. In a bid to find sympathetic ears he helped to organise a London-wide group for medics sharing similar political views. The group extended beyond doctors, attempting to involve nurses and other hospital workers. Sheila Rowbotham was of the opinion that he felt very isolated in the hospital world. It was not until later in that decade that coordinated action of hospital workers gathered speed. Widgery vented his frustrations dramatically.

In 1971, towards the end of his undergraduate years, Widgery wrote (or helped to write) a play entitled *The Doctor Show; A Radical Christmas Show*.[32] Contained within the script are a number of clues that shed light on Widgery's outlook on the medical world at this time. The front cover offers the following synopsis. 'The plot of this play is very slender. It concerns the entry into Medical School of an Innocent and his progress through disillusion to suicide. The play offers material to him and the

---

* Ian Smith was the leader of Rhodesia who declared the country independent from British rule during the 1960s. Critics believed that he delayed efforts to bring majority rule to the country.

audience to persuade him of the possibility of change.'

Widgery's view of medical school was not Utopian. One of the scenes is entitled 'Disillusion'. 'There were always exams, always consultants, always people coming up saying in their loud voices "You aren't working are you?" I watched myself sink into a world where the intellectual landscape was dominated by the Rugby Cup and what to wear to the hospital ball.'

It was a very different world for the boy who had not attended public school and whose parents had not gone to university. Within the play, statistics compiled by students of the Middlesex Hospital (now part of University College Hospital) are held up to the audience to demonstrate the problems with medical school admissions.

* A survey showed that 90% belonged to socioeconomic class I. Although in the general population 82% are classified as some grade of the working class, they provided only 5.6% of the Middlesex students.
* Individuals with a parent as a doctor, negligible in the general population, comprise 33% of all students at the Middlesex.
* A-level points required by the average student are from 9–12. But where a parent is a doctor, the average required slumped to 6–10 points. Lowest grades of all were required by those individuals (11.5% of the medical students) whose parent trained at the Middlesex.
* 65% of the medical students had been to a public or private school; these schools draw on 2.6% of the school-age population.

Within the environment of medical school, reflected in the play, we already see Widgery leaning towards general practice as the progressive alternative to hospital medicine. Hospital consultants are parodied in a scene entitled 'The Auction', set in a slave market selling pre-registration house officers.

And now the event of the sale. We are privileged to offer a model of unparallel excellence. Seven years' careful preparation and some of the best medical brains in the country have been concentrated into this one product. It always talked to the lecturer afterwards, always did extra work and always took extra exams. You always knew the right answers, didn't you? (Slave simpers.) Its friends were nothing but aides de camp of its ambition. Its life, its pleasures and its desires were all put second to its careerism ... This year's model comes with two papers in the *New England Journal of Medicine* already and a wide range of optional extras including the latest in blandishments, snobbery and gossip. It has absolutely no imagination.

Yes what am I offered? A consultant ... A Harley Street consultant with a big merit award.[32]

They are challenging words. Consultants are portrayed as somewhat narrow-minded. Work is everything, wider society far from their minds. It implies that they are simply out to further their own sense of self-importance and make money. This description is obviously a caricature but such depictions stem from something solid in the reality Widgery knew. In stark contrast to the hospital consultant is the general practitioner.

> Our first product is admittedly rather sub-standard but not without a certain period charm. It lacks clinical polish, its auscultation is – well – unreliable, and it has failed Pathology twice. (*Cough*). Nevertheless it's a friendly creature, has a real love for people and will wear well ... Yes, it has to be ... a GP.

We are also reminded that some GPs have been political. There is a scene where three students queue up to be humiliated by the consultant. In a manner of bedside teaching familiar to many, the consultant asks the student about the profession's great tradition. He reels off a list of names such as James Paget, Percival Pott, James Parkinson, Thomas Hodgkin, etc., and waits to be told about them.

> 'Well sir,' replies the student, 'I'm afraid I can't tell you much. I lose my memory when you ask me like that ... I think I read somewhere that Parkinson was a GP in Shoreditch who was active politically with the Chartists.'

This is an insult because you would not expect one of the 'profession's great traditions' to be a local community doctor. To be worthy of having a disease like Parkinson's named after you it would be more appropriate if the doctor were a physician or surgeon from a reputable London hospital. You certainly would not expect them to be mingling with subversives like the Chartists. The stage directions provided in the script, following the student's response, sum up these sentiments.

> Professor turns around the student's placard disgusted, it reads DUNCE.

Entering the East End

Thanks to such discontentment, it could be argued, Widgery ended up in the East End of London. 'The Dean of my medical school had decided to reward my insubordination and lassitude by exiling me to do house jobs in Shrewsbury. Instead I went through the London telephone directory's list of hospitals to solicit for alternatives. Bethnal Green Hospital was the first in the phone book and its hospital secretary told me to hop into a taxi, interviews were being held that morning.'[33]

It was at Bethnal Green that Widgery took his house jobs. There is a rather comical anecdote that illustrates the difficulty of trying to do the 'right thing' in the world of medicine. In the Accident and Emergency department, where Widgery was working at the time, there was a policy that when examining the homeless you should wear gloves. Because Widgery believed this to be inhumane and degrading, he conducted his clinical examinations gloveless. Sheila Rowbotham, with whom he was living at the time, remembers how on one occasion this backfired. A few days after one such examination, she and Widgery discovered they had contracted lice. Although they could not be certain of the causal link, they had strong suspicions. In the 1970s this was a serious public health issue. Chemists did not dispense lotions and combs; you had to attend a special council bath. Fuelling this embarrassment was the arrival of marked vans itching to fumigate their house. When the spray team saw all the books the intellectual couple possessed, they were adamant they had found the source of the head scratching.

After finishing his hospital jobs, Widgery entered general practice for the first time. Sheila Rowbotham got him a job with Dr Mike Leibson, having previously worked as his secretary. The practice would provide the crucial introduction to general practice in the East End.

> For five years I worked as an assistant to an elderly Jewish GP whose surgery was high over a chemist in Bethnal Green Road. Like many East-End GPs, he was a medical deviant fiercely independent, blunt to his patients who none the less admired him and relied on his skill and industry. He and I would have long philosophical arguments about art, politics and history in the Venus Steak House in our lunch hours. He would tell me about the imperfectability of human nature and reminisce about Bethnal Green in the days of the Krays.[34]*

Dr Leibson was an ex-member of the Communist Party. That he was also Jewish and an ex-army doctor made him something of an outsider within the medical profession. Sheila Rowbotham remembered him being 'completely amoral'. Leibson possessed a dark and cynical take on life, which was both endearing and challenging.† Nothing surprised him. It is difficult to appreciate what this experience was like. The kind of medicine being practised was very different from that found in health centres 20 years

---

* The Krays were notorious East-End gangsters who won mainly fear and some admiration from their local community.

† Rowbotham remembers how Dr Leibson 'would suddenly turn around and say, "What do you prefer, ecstasy or security?"' He wanted to know what you thought was better, a stable life or an exciting one.[28]

later. Clues are provided by his friends who attended as patients.

Nigel Fountain recounts, 'Leibson may have been fiercely defiant and blunt, but he was also fiercely invisible through his cloud of Number 6 cigarette smoke. I remember going into him and saying, "I've got this bump on my arm Dr Leibson." "Does it bother you?" "Not really". End of consultation.' David Phillips recalls another bemusing smoke-filled visit. 'I went as a patient. He'd say, "Have a fag, Dave, have a fag." We'd have a chat about politics, the health service, and all the time there'd be this waiting room full of people with God knows what terrible problems ... all I'd have was a sore throat.' Dr Paul Julian, a GP who was practising in the East End at this time, can understand the notion of smoking in front of patients; it was a way of demonstrating empathy.

Conditions and circumstances in Leibson's practice were tough. The premises were small and the medical team limited to one doctor and a receptionist. Women who had been badly beaten by their husbands in cases of domestic violence would turn up at the surgery. Since few alternatives existed, Leibson would give them £20 to check into a bed and breakfast for the night, thus escaping the husband.[35] Nor was it unheard of for a doctor to find a patient had been murdered, such was the fragility of their existence. This was the kind of frontline medicine being practised.

Leibson protected Widgery. Himself an outsider, he favoured the maverick. Not only that: he possessed ideologically sympathetic colleagues like the obstetrician Peter Huntingford, a pioneer of women's rights during birth. This inevitably made medicine more palatable to Widgery. It also meant that he had people fighting his corner if the more conservative started to question his wider actions.

By now Widgery was beginning to put aside his youthful ambition of becoming an orthopaedic surgeon. 'I think Dave knew he wasn't going to become a surgeon, because he knew he didn't do enough work to be a surgeon. By the time he got through fighting to get the qualifications to be a GP, I think for Widgery the prospect of going any further along this ladder meant that he would have to spend his entire life waging war on nine different fronts.'[20] Sheila Rowbotham also believes that, 'Widgery was not especially fired by medicine; he loved people but the subject matter could at times be rather dull.' Widgery's overriding ambition was to become a writer.

General practice allowed him to keep his politics and writing going. It also paid a wage, something his other interests did not. During the late 1970s and early 1980s Widgery did locum work in general practice. He worked regularly with Leibson and with Sam Smith, Markie Hayton and the St Stephen's Road Practice. He settled at Gill Street in 1985, having first discussed the issue with Anna Livingstone on a march in Trafalgar Square. He never sat any more exams; none were required.

As Widgery was discovering the joys of general practice, the flames that had sparked in 1968 were dying out. *Oz* had published its last issue in 1976 and many of those who had marched against Vietnam were now settling down to the pressing demands of family life and middle age. Not Widgery. The East End of London was a prime location for him to maintain his radical aspirations. A cosmopolitan area, ridden with poverty and pressing social issues, it fuelled Widgery's political life force.

Rock Against Racism

My skin has been burnt by the dry ice of James Baldwin's prose, my map of the world turned upside down by *The Black Jacobins*, my pulse set racing by Charlie Parker's assault on the Winter Palace of Jazz, tears brought to my boyish eyes by Miriam Makeba singing in the musical *King Kong*, my Marxism shaped by the encounters with the views of CLR James and WEB DuBois, and my Dalston Sundays slipstreamed by yearning, sublimely logical dub floating up from underneath the Cortinas.[36]

David Widgery

No one should have the right to tell anyone they can't live here because of the colour of their skin or their religion or whatever, the size of their nose. How could anyone vote for something so ridiculously inhumane?[37]

Johnny Rotten, Sex Pistols

In the late 1970s Widgery helped to found Rock Against Racism (RAR). This movement sprung up against the growing support for the racist National Front (NF) which was gathering support in East London. Racially motivated attacks were on the increase and immigrants were being blamed for other people's hardships. Ken Leech, a priest in the area, reflected on the rising tide. 'Between 1976–78 there was a marked increase in racist graffiti, particularly NF symbols, all over Tower Hamlets, and in the presence both of NF "heavies" and clusters of alienated young people at fascist locations, especially Bethnal Green.'[38] The NF was also winning increasing support in local elections.* The problem came to a head in 1978 when a young man, Altab Ali, was stabbed to death in Whitechapel. It was an unprovoked racist attack.

Aggravating the problem was music, a new kind of music which emerged around this time. The style became known as 'punk'. Roland Muldoon, Widgery's fellow cultural dissident, thought that the music was a good thing; by definition it was a form of political expression. 'The kids were

---

* The NF obtained a 19% share of the vote in Hackney South and Bethnal Green in 1976.

angry, they were making noise.' Widgery was not so certain. Renton, the socialist historian, explains why. 'NF members attempted to tap into this new punk style. They were helped by traces of ambiguity which punk displayed towards fascism. The style was anarchistic, but politically vague and individualistic ... Members of the Sex Pistols wore swastikas, as if the symbol could be a fashion statement, while one of their last singles pronounced that "Belsen Was A Gas".'[38]

In 1976 Eric Clapton, the famous guitarist, used a Birmingham concert to voice support for racist views expressed by the Conservative MP, Enoch Powell. For many this sounded wrong, especially since Clapton had become famous for doing his own version of a Bob Marley song. Red Saunders, a member of CAST, and Roger Huddle, a member of Islington IS branch, wrote the following letter:

> When we read about Eric Clapton's Birmingham concert when he urged support for Enoch Powell, we nearly puked. Come on Eric ... you've been taking too much of that *Daily Express* stuff and you know you can't handle it. Own up. Half your music is black. You're rock music's biggest colonist. You're a good musician but where would you be without the blues and R&B? You've got to fight the racist poison otherwise you degenerate into the sewer with the rats and all the money men who ripped off rock culture with their cheque books and plastic crap. We want to organise a rank and file movement against the racist poison in music. We urge support for Rock Against Racism. PS: Who shot the Sheriff, Eric? It sure as hell wasn't you![39]

The pair had the idea for a one-off anti-racist gig. When Widgery heard about it, he insisted on a far wider campaign. Music, politics, fighting racism ... it was his cultural cup of tea. Looking back at events in his book *Beating Time*, he wrote that:

> On one level Rock Against Racism was an orthodox anti-racist campaign simply utilising pop music to kick political slogans into the vernacular. But on another level, it was a jailbreak. We aimed to rescue the energy of Russian revolutionary art, surrealism and rock and roll from the galleries, the advertising agencies and the record companies and sue them again to change reality, as had always been intended. And have a party in the process.

RAR served to take the ambiguity away from punk music – 'Love music, hate racism.'

RAR had a fanzine, *Temporary Hoarding*, which allowed them to contribute to the debate through verbal and visual art. Widgery wrote many pieces for this and would be continually at work around the clock, with other members of the team, to get copies produced. In total 14 issues were published. Syd Shelton, the photographer who worked on the publication, said their average circulation was 25,000. Printed on A3 paper, they had music reviews, interviews with bands and satirical humour, but maintained a strong anti-racist theme. For example, in the second issue David Widgery interviewed Johnny Rotten, lead singer of the Sex Pistols, who became notorious for their anti-establishment single 'God Save the Queen'. While discussing whether or not punks need to wear safety pins through their noses, Widgery asks Rotten what he thinks about the Left, to which Johnny replies, 'It's fine talking about revolution. But that's all they tend to do. They are too separated from reality. Don't get into the people they are trying to involve. It comes across as a condescending attitude which isn't appreciated.' Widgery and his friends were trying to break down this political perception.

Temporary Hoarding was full of bold and daring stuff. For example, it campaigned against issues of policing, like the SUS laws, which meant people could be arrested if suspected of loitering with intent to steal. The police tended to be more suspicious of black people than white – a mechanism of racial prejudice was allowed to perpetuate. Widgery also took time to challenge homophobic attitudes, which were very common in reggae music. Then he would slip in something about why he thought capitalism was bad. 'You're just as miserable whether you buy the product or not. It's not in their interest for you ever to reach the goal of contentment. It's always got to be one step beyond, there's always a more sophisticated hi-fi, a more exotic holiday for you to feel dissatisfied with the one you just bought. If you ever became content you wouldn't want to buy anymore.'

The formation of the Anti-Nazi League (ANL) in 1977 fed into the RAR movement. Concerts were organised up and down the country. While there were many people involved, David Widgery is perceived to have been the central figure. Energy and enthusiasm defined him. Red Saunders was always impressed by his ability to mobilise people. He possessed a knack for mass appeal. Days prior to the Manchester RAR Carnival very few tickets had been sold. 'After persistent pestering Widgery managed to get The Clash to agree to play... Word got around that they were on the bill and tickets sold rapidly.'[40]

Despite its socialist underpinning you did not have to hold Marxist ideals to think fighting racism was a good thing. While some were marching because they were tired of having friends attacked, some were attending because they liked the music. The message's medium was crucial. A rock band drumming home anti-racism carried more weight than someone speaking earnestly, wearing brown corduroy trousers, in a half-empty room.

The three great carnivals put on by RAR, Victoria Park, Brockwell Park and Belle Vue, Manchester, were extraordinary moments of popular protest. And while the Anti-Nazi League organisation in the trade unions was ideologically effective as counter-propaganda, the people mobilised on the demonstrations and the pickets were the younger people coming to anti-racism and anti-fascism through the 'moral' perspectives offered by Rock Against Racism and the popular music culture.[41]

Raphael Samuel, a socialist historian, described the Victoria Park concert, 1978, as 'the most working class demonstration I have been on, and one of the very few of my adult lifetime to have sensibly changed the climate of public opinion'.[42] The event attracted 80 000 people. David Renton, one of the few people to write about this movement, considers it to have been one of the largest of its kind in Britain. 'Between 1977 and 1979, at least nine million ANL leaflets were distributed and 750 000 badges sold. Fifty local Labour Parties affiliated, along with 30 AUEW branches, 25 trade councils, 13 shop stewards committees, 11 NUM lodges, and similar numbers of branches from the TGWU, CPSA, TASS, NUJ, and NUPE.'[42] The result was a direct attack on racist sentiment and racist organisations. NF 'activists were unable to put their message across, their graffiti were painted out, and they could not march'.

RAR was not without its critics. For many on the left, RAR was not political enough. One activist lamented that, 'there wasn't enough politics talked to the audience'. At the same time, according to some in the music world, it was too political. RAR had the power to make or break bands based on their ideology. A rift exists in the SWP about the significance of RAR. Some claim Widgery exaggerated its role and that it was really the ANL who should claim the credit. For others the ANL and RAR were in many ways synonymous. The distinction made between the two organisations, as Renton explains, was not simply a question of personal bickering. 'David Widgery, Red Saunders, Ruth Gregory and Syd Shelton hoped to use RAR to generate a new political language, less verbal and more visual, more youthful and populist than the socialism which they inherited.' RAR eventually petered out, with events like Live Aid taking its place. In the early 1980s there were some Rock Against Thatcher (RAT) concerts organised. RAT did not last long.

If all this seems like small print we should not forget the bigger picture. Throughout his life Widgery fought against racism. He would challenge and engage people. He would try and find out why they held such sentiments and try to persuade them otherwise. Widgery believed that most racists were not hardened fascists but people who had arrived at their views as a result of unemployment and deprivation. The journalist Darcus Howe spoke at a memorial meeting for David Widgery. He had brought up five children in Britain. 'The first four had grown up angry, fighting racism forever around them. The fifth child,' he said, 'had grown up "black at ease".' Why had this been possible with the fifth child? Darcus attributed her 'space' to the ANL in general and to David Widgery in particular.[43]

Dark ages/1980s/the Hackney resident

Mrs T will grant us freedom not to have any obligation towards fellow human beings who are ill, out of work, or incapable so that we have the freedom to select what private ward, public school dorm, restaurant or town house we wish for ourselves ... This morally squalid equation of freedom with the thickness of your wallet is still more horrible a formula when you consider that it can only be achieved by a deliberate campaign to make the poor poorer. Mrs T's much-loved 'scroungers' who are present hanging onto their dignity by their teeth and finger-nails, will be formally and legally kicked over the edge. For their own good of course, because Mrs Thatcher's new brand of Toryism knows that misfortune is but the evidence of vice, weakness or error, and that it is therefore kind to be cruel.[44]

David Widgery

Despite Widgery's efforts Margaret Thatcher and the Conservatives were elected to power in 1979. During the subsequent years, public services were neglected in favour of private enterprise. Society, Thatcher said, did not exist. For the Left it must have been a nightmare come true; optimism evaporated and pessimism prevailed. Amongst the down-trodden faces Widgery remained upbeat. 'As for our Left, bedraggled but alive, we are still infants. We have not yet come of age and are far from the heights of our powers. But we survived and, in Tom Mann's words, intend to grow more dangerous as we grow old.'[45]

It was not quite the revolution Widgery had hoped for. National mass movements, let alone international mass movements, were few and far between. Widgery was never again to organise anything as big as RAR or to see marches like those against the Vietnam War. The 1980s saw Widgery defined as something of an enthusiastic Hackney local resident.

Widgery helped revive the Hackney Literary and Philosophical Society (where Richard Smith, future editor of the *BMJ*, came to talk about ill health and poverty) and started the Hackney Men's Group, a group of males who would meet regularly, drink beer and discuss their sexuality. When Roland Muldoon needed some theatrical assistance, Widgery was more than happy to help.

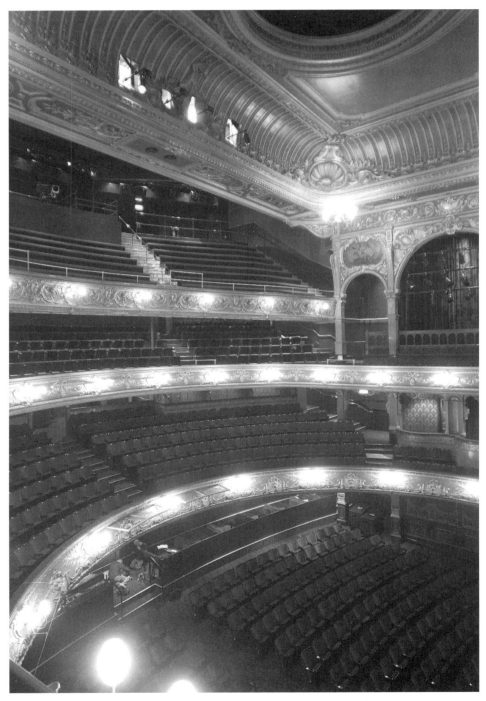

The Hackney Empire – the theatre Widgery loved. It gave the local population a landmark to be proud of.

Having stopped touring Britain, Muldoon had taken on the running of the Hackney Empire Theatre in 1986. An old East-End music hall, it had been lying derelict as an old Mecca Bingo. Widgery was an important ally.

> When we got to the Hackney Empire, it was inevitable that I suggest he be on the Board. And the reason we wanted him on the Board is because we had to pack it with left-wing people. So if ever there was a coup … We had no money whatsoever, and we were complete-left wing pirates … having Widgery on the Board, because he was a doctor, might be a bit more respectable.[46]

In *New Society* Widgery commemorated its first year of survival. He sung its tale of discovery and pointed to its attributes of being run by a non-commercial management. Above all it was something for the local community.

> Hackney itself is the same inner-urban mess of desolation. Poverty, rowdiness and HGVs and the Empire won't change that. But it has given a new pride, élan and a sense of possibility to the borough. At the first annual general meeting last month there was much anguishing about the mistakes and the scale of the fund-raising challenge (the first £50 000 is now needed in four months). But a commercial management would have been patting itself on the back if it had achieved a tenth of what the Empire's team have done in just a year. Harry the doorman seemed to think it was very simple. A great theatre is lit again. And the volunteer who operates the follow-spot thought the same sort of thing. 'All I know is that I see a lot of heads. There's grey and bald and dread-locks. But they all love being here.'[47]

There was rarely a moment when Widgery was not writing or campaigning. His interest in the health and politics of the community he served developed in a new way. As Sue Collinson, a family friend, reflected, 'I remember when David had to make that decision to enter general practice full time, because he was just doing locums here and there. When he got embedded in his own practice, with his own cohort of patients, he became enormously committed to that group of people, and became I think a gentler person. He had a lot of hard edges at the beginning of the 1980s. He became a lot more human.'

If it affected his patients, it affected him. The construction of Canary Wharf and the Docklands, which epitomised the 1980s, was bitterly opposed. He believed it would erode the community of the East End, driving local people away and replacing them with a nine-to-five business community.

Settling down with Juliet Ash and her son, family life was fast becoming a reality. But with such reality sadly came great tragedy. In 1982 his first daughter, Molly, died of Rhesus haemolytic disease soon after her birth. Without any question the event was devastating, but if anyone was going to find a small ideological consolation it was Widgery.

> Molly was born and so nearly lived only because of a chain of unselfish human beings which stretched from the unknown blood donors whose gifts sustained her in the womb to the nurses who got Molly and us through so many nights and still spared a thought to tuck a white carnation in her death wraps. In the 1980s, politically dominated by the philosophy of possessive individualism, the NHS still allows a different set of values to flourish. And it makes manifest the spirit of human solidarity which is at the core of socialism, and which our present rulers are so concerned to eradicate. While Molly's death is a tragedy, her life was something brave and marvellous.[48]

While previously his focus might have been elsewhere, general practice became more central to his life. As Ruth Gregory noted, 'He had a romantic view of being a writer. Like I might have about being an artist. He made a definite change in his involvement with being a GP. And began to concentrate more. And began to really enjoy it as well. I don't think he really did enjoy it so much up until then. He became involved in the area.' Medicine in the East End became an expression of his politics, during a climate when many people believed the causes of the Left to be dead. Collinson believes that, 'Rolling up his sleeves and helping people one to one became a substitute for a more globally active position. I think he increasingly withdrew. Obviously with the birth of his daughters, family became more important. Work and family became his world. Although he remained politically and intellectually active, his *activism* subsided.' In the early 1990s Widgery reflected that 'being radical today is about fighting to keep hold of what we already have. I used to think it was going around with a red flag and berets, but it's not been that for the last 15–20 years . . . To hold the ground and fight for aluminium frames, meals on wheels and high blood pressure screening in the present context is pretty damn revolutionary.'[49]

It was the NHS and issues relating to health that were at the forefront of Widgery's actions and writings, the real focus of this book. The range of activities he engaged in relating to health was immense. By the early 1990s he had become a well-established voice within the medical profession, thanks largely to his regular column in the *BMJ*. In 1991 he was due to embark on a one-year sabbatical as a fellow of the Wellcome Institute for the History of Medicine. He had been commissioned to write a history of medicine in the East End. It was never written. David Widgery died in September 1992. He was 45.

Chapter 4

Medical reasoning

When people talk about doctors being artists, it's nearly always due to the shortcomings of society. In a better society, in a juster one, the doctor would be much more of a pure scientist.[50]

John Sassall

Being a doctor is to have done well in the game of life. It is the Rolls Royce/Jaguar/Mercedes of occupations. Sit back, turn up the music and soak up the respect, admiration and jealousy. Happiness is just around the corner. Follow your dreams. Let art and science melt in your mouth to become Renaissance Woman/Man. With an endless cocktail of knowledge to keep your mind refreshed (and validated), could there be any other reason to practise medicine?

Wait. I think we might have missed something – the point. Isn't there something that unites all health professionals? That's it. I remember it now – 'the fundamental desire to help other human beings'. (Be careful of saying this aloud though. It can make you look naive and idealistic.)

When you peel away the cynicism and pessimism, the radiating core remains: doctors get great satisfaction from helping others. 'It is one of the most beautiful compensations of this life that no man can sincerely try to help another without helping himself.'[51] The reality of this is sadly not quite so uplifting. A psychiatrist reminded me of this. In one of many conversations we had during a clinic where DNA (Did Not Arrive) was the most popular entry in the notes, he had the strength of mind to analyse the world of a training doctor. 'You are a strange bunch. Whilst others relaxed at A-level you were working hard; no one ever admits they are working hard – that is strange in itself; you put yourselves through what is essentially a barbaric macho system. You cut up dead bodies and are not expected to bat an eyelid. You show no emotion in situations full of pain and suffering. Who would want to do such a thing?'

The world of the qualified doctor appears no less strange than that of the unqualified. In 2001 Richard Smith, editor of the *BMJ*, asked why so many doctors are unhappy.

'The most obvious cause of doctors' unhappiness' Smith argued, 'is that they feel overworked and undersupported. They hear politicians make extravagant promises but then must explain to patients why the health service cannot deliver what is promised. Endless initiatives are announced, but on the ground doctors find that operating lists are cancelled, they cannot admit or discharge patients, and community services are disappearing. They struggle to respond, but they feel as though they are battling the system rather than being supported by it.'[52]

Not all doctors are unhappy but virtually everyone admits to having their happiness tested. One doctor, in response to Smith's editorial, encouraged people to think of the positives, like saving people's lives, but lamented, 'The pace of change in the United Kingdom is daunting and unmanageable. A plethora of clinical guidelines, frameworks and targets to meet is too much when doctors are expected to continue their day-to-day clinical work. As much as I enjoy my work, I find myself utterly exhausted with the long hours, the extra management time, the lack of support from senior colleagues and the battering by the press and politicians. The impact of my work on family life is too often unacceptable.'[53]

In 1967, John Berger, in *A Fortunate Man*, described the medical profession as 'the most idealised of professions. Yet it is idealised abstractedly. Some of the young who decide to become doctors are at first influenced by this ideal. But I would suggest that one of the fundamental reasons why so many doctors become cynical and disillusioned is precisely because, when the abstract idealism has worn thin, they are uncertain about the value of the patients they are treating. This is not because they are callous or personally inhuman: it is because they live in and accept a society which is incapable of knowing what a human life is worth.' Trends in medicine would seem to amplify this sentiment. Are patients simply commodities and health professionals machines? If so, it would seem to perpetuate sorrow. In a *BMJ* web survey on reasons for doctors' unhappiness, being 'left picking up the pieces in a society that has lost ways of coping with pain, sickness and death' was a high scorer.[54]

Doctors have to make sense of things that seem unjust and unfair. The answers cannot be found in textbooks. Despite being frequently responsible, molecules are never accountable. Going to work sends a doctor spiralling towards questions most would rather forget. They can be medical – 'What is the current level of random blood glucose for which a glucose tolerance test is recommended?' They can be ethical – 'Do I ask this girl about contraception in front of her mother or try and speak to her on her own?' They can be metaphysical – 'The appointment system … how does that work?' They can also be social – 'How are Mrs Jones and her family ever going to feel well, living in this horrible, damp and overcrowded flat?'

The social in medicine is important, more important than we perhaps give it credit. 'Ah,' the contrarian says, 'but if science were concerned with the social, it would cease to be a science, it would become a social science'. This is not a matter of linguistic nicety. Doctors would rather think about the blood glucose level than the life circumstances of a patient. The reasons are straightforward. More often than not, science is relatively simple and quick, while the social takes time and energy; the outcome of one's actions cannot be readily measured. Happiness is Prozac. So perhaps I should rephrase my earlier statement. 'The social is more important than we are *able* to give it credit for.'

Social factors in medicine are messy. Like people begging in the streets, they stare us in the face, but we would rather turn away. Occasionally our conscience can override our sense of awkwardness. You try and do something. It helps the person at the time, but a week later you see the same person in the same situation. Nevertheless you keep up the effort. A couple of emotionally draining years down the line, you realise that your colleagues stopped caring long ago. In fact some of them never cared at all. They finish before you, they look healthier than you, they seem happier than you. What a harsh world we live in. You try and do the right thing but the world kicks sand in your face.

Poverty and ill health

Literature is filled with anecdotal examples of how poverty goes hand in hand with poor health. The following is an extract from Dostoevsky's *Crime and Punishment*, where poverty, illness and crime seem inextricably linked. A young woman, who has been forced to prostitute herself in order to feed her children, is being defended from accusations of theft, by someone similarly destitute.

> 'Oh dear! You are fools, fools,' she cried, addressing the whole room, 'you don't know what a heart she has, what a girl she is! She take it, she? She'd sell her last rag, she'd go barefoot to help you if she needed it, that's what she is! She has the yellow passport because my children were starving, she sold herself for us!' ... The wail of the poor, consumptive, helpless woman seemed to produce a great effect on her audience. The agonised, wasted, consumptive face, the parched blood-stained lips, the hoarse voice, the tears unrestrained as a child's, the trustful, childish and yet despairing prayer for help were so piteous that everyone seemed to feel for her.[55]

Such observations correlate with more methodical evidence. In late 18th- and early 19th-century Paris, enlightened men of science set about uncovering the truth. Patients, generally the poor and destitute, were observed whilst ill. The doctors tapped and listened, they prodded and probed, they searched for clues and patterns. When life left the patients, they dissected them. They correlated signs and symptoms with the state of the internal organs, deducing, for example, that the coughing of blood might mean something miliary was happening in the lungs.*

This desire to count and correlate was something that extended beyond the confines of the hospitals. The story of René Louis Villermé, one of the first to investigate the relationship between health and society, is described in Roy Porter's *The Greatest Benefit to Mankind*.

> Analysing the differential mortality among the Paris arrondissements (districts), and testing all the conventional environmental factors such as altitude, soil and climate, he found none explained the mortality patterns. Likewise with overcrowding: no clear correlations emerged.
>
> Having exhausted the morbific determinants dear to Enlightenment physicians, Villermé tried economic status. Eureka! The poorest arrondissements consistently showed highest mortality levels. The rue de la Mortellerie, packed like sardines with *les misérables*, had a death rate of 30.6 per thousand, while a stone's throw away amongst the richer residents of the quais of the Ile-Saint-Louis it was less than two thirds as high. The rich lived longer; the poor bore, and lost, more children and died young. In later studies of the textile industry, Villermé confirmed these conclusions in life-tables for the working class, correlating mortality against income. Poverty and illness went together.[56]

Medicine has travelled many miles since then. Antibiotics, operations which (quite crucially) patients survive, clinical research, mass vaccinations, batch orders of white coats, and – before we or history realised it – the present was here. So great are the achievements (we have cured so many things that once seemed impossible) that we crane our necks, trying hard to catch a glimpse of the future. Well done – but what about this relationship between poverty and ill health?

Inequalities in Health was published in 1980.[57] The inquiry was chaired by Sir Douglas Black and became known as *The Black Report*. The report described how inequalities in health were directly related to inequalities in society. The Conservative government of the day, 'whose plans were different and decisive',[58] tried to limit the impact of the publication by publishing a small number of copies on an August bank holiday. It was perceived as a cover-up, which unsurprisingly only fuelled interest. Penguin published copies of the report and news of its contents quickly

---

* The classic appearance of TB is a chest x-ray with diffuse white spots, said to look like millet seed.

spread.[59] Brian Able Smith had pointed out, just prior to the report's publication, that 'despite 30 years of the National Health Service, mortality rates between social classes are if anything getting wider rather than narrower. These are problems which need intensive investigation and remedial action in whatever field that can be effective.'[60] *The Black Report* showed that people living in conditions associated with bad housing, unemployment, poverty, etc., were far more likely to suffer poor health. 'The association was universal. Wherever there was social disparity there was disparity in health, and disparity was to be found in a wide range of conditions from obesity to accident rates, arthritis and stroke.'[59]

Critics of these findings point out that they are relative, that the poor are not like the people Dickens portrayed. At the same time, the relative differences between rich and poor remain disturbing. If we are to believe a follow-up study to *The Black Report*, inequalities in healthcare and society are getting worse. This second report leaves no question as to the required action. 'The key policy that will reduce inequalities in health is the alleviation of poverty through the reduction in income and wealth inequality. Poverty can be reduced by raising the standards of living of poor people through increasing their incomes. The costs would be borne by the rich and would reduce inequalities overall.'[61]

For medical professionals especially, life can seem too busy to think of politics and social inequalities, let alone of ways to address them. Certainly it is not encouraged. My own recent experience as a medical student serves to illustrate the point. As in any responsible medical school, the clinical pathology course included a lecture on tuberculosis. The number one cause for contracting the disease is poverty. 'But,' says the clinical pathology lecturer, 'that's not for us to worry about. We'll leave that to the politicians.'

It would be strange if all doctors had ignored social issues like poverty, if every member of the 'caring profession' had folded their arms and said, 'Sorry, would love to help, but no can do. My job is medicine; politics is someone else's. Blame the manager or the system.' Widgery could not leave politics to the politicians. He was a socialist, and his socialism was fuelled by medicine.

Healthcare according to need rather than wealth is not just a good moral principle. It has been shown to work. And to be more efficient and effective than the commercial-based medical sector in North America. This is ground which must be held against governments who make no secret of their wish to return to the old two-tier medical care of charity and minimal medicine for the majority with a lucrative private sector providing VIP care to those who can foot the bills.

But if I ever get complacent about what can be achieved by medical measures alone, I need only go as far as I did this lunchtime: to the local supermarket. There I will almost certainly know half a dozen shoppers and will be able to see the trolleys quaking with pop and sugar, cheap cosmetics and ciggies: not because my patients are bad people. But because those products are cheap and filling and quick and keep the kiddies quiet. And it's then, not in the consulting room, that I renew my practical and intellectual commitment to social change.[62]

Widgery was not the first 'radical' to share similar sentiments. Che Guevara started life as a medical student. Rudolf Virchow, the founding father of modern cellular pathology, spoke of things other than thrombotic triads. He stated that, 'medicine is a social science, and politics is nothing more than medicine on a large scale'.[63] In Britain, the Socialist Medical Association (SMA) helped draw up the plans that were used to create the NHS. They argued passionately in arenas believed to be beyond the scope of medicine. For example, during the 1930s, with fascism creeping across Europe, the SMA spoke out. They believed it to be 'against the universal spirit that has developed in the medical profession during past centuries'.[64]

For some, however, Widgery's socialism and his medical career must have appeared a contradiction. During the 1960s and 1970s medicine came under increasing criticism. People pointed out that medicine was not all good. Some believed that to become a doctor was to collude with the enemy, namely the state. 'The Great Concern about the apparent ineffectiveness of medicine in solving our health problems seems to ignore the fact that the main function of medicine in present-day capitalism is not to solve/cure but take care of and administer the diswelfare that is created by the social relations of production.'[65]

One of the questions people on the left asked was, 'What is the most valuable position I can take up within society to help the socialist struggle?' Anna Livingstone, a partner of Widgery's at the Limehouse practice and a committed socialist, graduated from Oxford with an arts degree in 1971. She seriously considered becoming a truck driver before deciding on medicine, such was the political atmosphere at the time. Michael Rosen explained the thinking. 'In the Marxist tradition, the most decent thing to be doing is to be a male labourer within the hierarchy. The idea is that the real power lies in the working classes where the revolution might happen. The most valuable thing you can do, if a member of one of these political parties, is to be a member of the organised working class.'[14]

It is difficult to say whether Widgery seriously thought about these criticisms of the medical profession. Part of him simply thought that being a doctor was a decent thing to be doing. After all, modern medicine had saved his life. This might explain why for someone so radical he could be perceived as conservative. For example, he had no time for RD Laing's criticisms of the psychiatry profession. Nor would he ever waste breath advocating homeopathy. Instead he preferred the authority of the expert medical opinion.

On the other hand, being an East-End GP and defending the NHS was hardly playing to the stereotypes of medical power. Nor did he shy away from criticising the profession. In 1979 Widgery wrote, 'The British Medical Association (not unfairly known as the Tory Party at the bedside) still end their chapter on "Ethics" with the advice that "when all is said and done, a chap knows what's cricket".'[66] This put distance between him and the image of a Harley Street consultant with pinstriped suit, top hat and cane.

Michael Rosen defended Widgery when an ideological incompatibility was suggested. 'He wasn't going to take any shit from people who said he was middle class or a sell out or anything like that. People who had slaved away in the docks and were now in a lonely flat with a broken back, any help he could give to those people would be worthwhile. It wasn't charity. It was paid for ... Part of development in IS thinking was to appreciate that other layers get drawn into being oppositional in a time of crisis. This is obvious in education, also the NHS.'[14]

To be a GP on the front line was to be out there. This was profoundly important. It meant that Widgery could engage people in politics, that he was involved in the local community of the East End. Such sentiment is reflected in the writing of his political hero Peter Sedgwick, the following quote having appeared in the introduction to Widgery's book *The Left in Britain*.*

Workers are particularly suspicious of people from Marxist groups who show up only when there is some excitement at the factory in the form of a strike, and are nowhere to be seen during the many periods, some of them amounting to years, when the activity of the working class falls short of open strike action. Nor can one play the part of the adept servitor of trade unionism, the technician of facts and figures who just happens to have more time to do research for the shop floor. The Socialist must join the workers' movement as a trade unionist in his own right, with card, rule-book and box of anti-management tricks, undergoing the same problems of skill and morale in leadership as those he is addressing. His politics must be open: not regurgitated by the yard into every resolution with a practical content but visible to everyone, displayed on his lapel rather than tucked away behind it.

---

* Widgery wrote of Sedgwick, 'Almost unique amongst many Marxist intellectuals of the 1956 vintage, he didn't just write about the left but he made it.'[67]

A political GP

A number of images spring to mind when we think about the GP. Maybe it is the reassuring face of a doctor at the bedside, looking down at a patient who has by now become a good family friend. Or perhaps it is the sound of a telephone ringing in the early hours of the morning. Moments later, ignoring the protests of loved ones, the doctor plunges gallantly into the deep and mysterious night on another home visit.*

Fundamentally the GP's role necessitates the care of patients in close proximity to the local community. Scientific universals are important but the true connective tissue is found in patients' lives. Travel up and down the country and you will witness the geographical variation of the doctor–patient encounter. Sleep loss as a result of sheep loss was probably higher in those areas affected by the 2001 foot-and-mouth crisis. No doctor (or health professional for that matter) can practise on a daily basis without becoming aware of the wider community they serve. No surgeon can operate at the Royal London Hospital without realising that a large Bangladeshi population lives in Whitechapel. No consultant can work in Colchester without knowing that the town has a large army barracks. You might simply say this is a truism – local people possess local knowledge. The difference is that health professionals, especially GPs, have to incorporate social variations into their daily practice. If the area in which you work is ridden with social problems, it is impossible to exist in oblivion.

This is where the political nature of medicine lies and what led Iona Heath to argue that GPs were political by definition. Their default exposure to the community they serve, by way of their daily interaction with patients, means that they cannot help but formulate an opinion about the state of society. She cites the example of voting patterns in general elections to reinforce her point. Despite their traditional Conservative following, the majority of doctors were in favour of a Labour government in 1992, five years before the Conservatives were defeated. GPs were aware that the NHS was not being looked after. While doctors may be predisposed to thinking about politics, few are as explicitly political. David Widgery was a doctor not afraid to display his politics firmly on his lapel.

---

* Since Widgery's time this has been replaced by a less personalised system (but less strenuous on the doctor) called the GP Co-operative, where doctors from different practices pool their responsibilities to share the responsibilities of 'on calls'.

Chapter 5

Changing reality

Healthcare, for Widgery, was a metaphor for much that was wrong in the world. As was quoted at the outset, 'My own life, as much as my politics, tells me that the levels of compassion with which a society treats its sick and crippled, its old and its feeble-minded, is the real measure of that society's level of civilisation.'[68] By the mid-1980s Widgery's main focus was medicine. As we touched on earlier, this was partly due to the activities he had previously associated himself with, like *Oz* and RAR, diminishing. Nevertheless, medical practice was still an expression of David Widgery's political ideology and this chapter aims to look at how the two related.

Documentary evidence

Limehouse Doctor was a fly-on-the-wall documentary made about David Widgery shortly before his death. Filmed in the surgery, in patients' homes, in the car between visits, it provides a good glimpse of what his daily life as a GP was like. We find him continually soliciting on behalf of his patients, seeking symptomatic relief from problems whose origins are found in wider society. Simply doing his job was an important means of shaking up the system and tackling inequalities.

In one instance Widgery visits a Bangladeshi couple with two children who are being evicted from their council flat. All the residents in the block are being moved to make way for a business development. The husband is a mature student struggling to find work. The wife speaks no English and is chronically depressed. No single tablet will cure their problems but that does not mean the doctor is powerless. Widgery speaks persuasively on the phone with the consultant psychiatrist; a well-drafted letter might help the family's case with the housing department. Later on we see the family being forced into temporary accommodation. The wife is deteriorating, the husband becoming increasingly distraught at their predicament. The prospects do not look good.

In another scene Widgery attempts to find a respite bed for an elderly man who is chronically ill. The bed is intended to provide his wife with a break from the strain of constant care. Widgery explains for the camera that funding cuts in the NHS have meant that this service has been scrapped. We see him on the phone attempting to negotiate a bed for the man. This time his endeavours prove successful. We are left wondering if someone less persistent and determined would have achieved a similar result. There are numerous scenes like this in the documentary, with a common theme. If the social circumstances of these patients were not so bad, if there were better levels of healthcare provision, the health and lives of the patients would improve.

These are things that many GPs and hospital doctors, from their daily experience with patients, know only too well. But the degree to which the social is deemed relevant by the doctor will always vary. Some may dwell on the social context more (or less) than others. For example, it is not unusual for doctors to minimise the housing issue, seeing it as a problem they are powerless to effect. Similarly, there may be those who care, but find it necessary to ignore the social simply to continue functioning. Cruel as it may be, there may be some doctors who really do not care. Widgery considered it one of his overriding responsibilities as a GP. To socialists, he was redistributing resources in a working-class area. To others, he was simply a conscientious doctor.

We should also note that Widgery was very taken aback by what he saw as a GP. During the 1980s many believed that he underwent something of a process of realisation. Instead of thinking, 'Ah, drug addicts, what great people', he changed to a more, 'Ah, drug addicts, how tiresome they can be, robbing and stealing, being a nuisance in the surgery.'[*] Dr Trevor Turner remembers how he and Widgery would discuss chronic alcoholics, suggesting he should get them to take cannabis instead.[†] How successful such endeavours were we shall never know.

It does not take an expert to point out that such tactics have limitations. Hustling at an individual level is necessary but somewhat paradoxical. Services are limited and demand high, especially in areas of deprivation: by helping one patient you are probably denying someone equally needy. This is why Widgery invested energy engaging in the politics of health provision.

---

[*] Anecdote given by Sue Collinson, friend of David Widgery and partner of Trevor Turner.
[†] Due to the illegality of the substance it would be impossible to conduct a clinical trial.

Meeting wider issues

Traditionally, GPs are more autonomous than most health professionals. Running practices as small businesses, they make decisions about how to spend their money. Every practice is a plethora of choice epitomised by gatherings like the partners' and practice meetings. The problems tackled can vary from the mundane ('Should we buy a Fairer Trade brand of coffee?') to the more profound ('Do we expand reception or employ an additional nurse?'). Politics is everywhere. The doctors at Gill Street Health Centre, where Widgery became a partner, shared socialist ideals. Trevor Turner points out that it needed SWP members to encourage Widgery into the world of medicine more permanently. 'By working with them he could think "I'm working for the SWP and being a doctor, I'm not just taking the money".' Gill Street was not the kind of practice to sacrifice smaller list sites for more money, nor would they object to Anti-Nazi League posters being displayed. Surprisingly, this was not the most radical practice around. Staff at the Hoxton Health Collective received exactly the same wage, doctors, nurses, receptionists and cleaners included.

Towards the 1990s, general practice was going though a particularly turbulent patch. The 1990 GP contract, which introduced the internal market and set targets for cervical screening and immunisation, was introduced against popular opinion.[69] In the documentary, filmed in a practice meeting, we see Widgery lamenting the time it takes to do a cervical smear. His complaint is that there is not enough time to do all these things, let alone more. In a bid to limit government changes Widgery got involved with organisations outside the practice.

David Widgery was a keen and active member of the North East London Local Medical Committee (LMC), the main negotiating body for GPs in Hackney, Tower Hamlets and Newham. Widgery was also a member of the Medical Practitioners Union (MPU) – dragging Trevor Turner along to the meetings. Widgery was therefore working for better provision for the wider population, not simply the patient in front of him. When the Royal London was deciding whether or not to become a hospital trust, a self-governing body, it was Widgery who proposed a ballot of the local GPs. There was a fear that business interests would distract from health needs. Ninety-four per cent of GPs opposed the formation of a trust.

In *Limehouse Doctor*, we see Widgery attending the GP Forum, a meeting of local doctors. He explains for the camera, 'The most important thing the NHS did in East London was to stop GPs being commercial rivals.' This is a statement against the introduction of fund holding, which he believed would make the service more fragmented. 'You don't want patients flocking to one practice thinking they can get a better deal.' The GP Forum is meeting to ensure that doctors agree upon the services they want to provide and to try to limit the corrosive effects they believe competition will bring.

If there was a meeting happening in East London you could bet that Widgery would be there. According to Anna Livingstone, 'When these groups met, Dave was a powerful asset. His political awareness and historical background, combined with his gift of the gab, meant he could be very persuasive.'* Widgery was something of a beacon to which other East-End doctors looked. If you thought general practice was getting a rough deal, that services were being eroded, that the extent of deprivation in East London was being ignored, that government changes seemed senseless, and if you considered yourself a bit of a lefty, then it was probably wonderful to know David Widgery was fighting your corner.

Different disciplines think in different ways. This was the case when Widgery sat on the Consultants Liaison Committee at the Royal London Hospital. He was furious at the proposal to build a helipad that would cover major traumas within the M25. Costing millions, the project symbolised high-tech medicine removed from the local community. Widgery believed the money would be better invested in projects directly benefiting the surrounding population. Although unsuccessful in his endeavours, he showed himself not to be a person who preached only to the converted.

There is nothing extraordinary about what Widgery was doing. He pursued channels open to all GPs. What was special is that he possessed the energy and strength of his convictions to explore them. Most people do not. There are many good reasons why this is so. Life is complicated enough. There is no guarantee that you will reach your destination. What happens if you feel you are getting nowhere? What if traditional tactics don't work? One medical emergency in particular demonstrated that David Widgery was not afraid to try something different.

Keeping hospitals alive

Early on New Year's morning, a docker arriving with a child with a badly scalded hand took a swing at the gate porter who had to tell him that Casualty had been closed at midnight that night, for good. . . . When

---

* 'He was a wonderful speaker, whether on beat poetry, the NHS, Mayakovsky, punk or opera.'[7]

your kid is screaming with pain, you can't cope with 'shadow regional health authorities' and 'formal recommendations to the Secretary of State'. You just know that one more of the handful of amenities provided for East-London workers is gone. And you lash out ... A man outside the closed Casualty with a hand dripping with blood who, surprisingly good-naturedly, offered to sign a protest petition in his own haemoglobin, said, 'Well, unless they start knocking down the estates and selling them for firewood, there's nothing much else down this way they can close, is there?'[70]

David Widgery

The 1970s represented a loss of innocence for the health service. People were living longer, the cost of medical treatment was rising and, to make matters worse, the global markets were in oily turmoil. Government faced tough economic decisions. Hospital building plans, which had looked feasible in 1968, had to be rethought, with London coming under particular scrutiny. The capital had a disproportionate number of acute hospital services in relation to the rest of the country. Labour adopted a policy of financial relocation from the South East to the North of Britain. The Resource Allocation Working Party (RAWP) was announced in July 1975.[71]

Looking back during the late 1980s, Widgery stated that he was not opposed to the principle. 'The concept of redistribution was, and is, entirely right. Indeed it was the Left which insisted on drawing attention to the inequalities in regional spending within the NHS.'[72] However, as the *BMJ* put it, 'The fundamental objection to RAWP can be stated in one sentence; when resources are growing reallocation can be more equitable, but in a period of recession it makes hardship worse. The regions who receive more money through RAWP are not getting more money, just fewer cuts.'[73]

In 1977 David Widgery was a junior casualty officer in Bethnal Green Hospital. The experience convinced him that the service performed an important social role.

The Casualty Departments also have to deal with patients who are homeless, unregistered with a GP or not bothered to attend, as well as their bona fide emergencies and ambulance work. So a casualty officer's job becomes more and more like that of a receiving officer under the old Poor Law. He or she has to balance a medical assessment against the patient's home circumstances and the relatives' resources. The casualty officer stands at the collision point between the patient's need, the family's worries and the hospital's overcrowded beds. How often have I searched a patient for an upturning big toe or a possible mass in the rectum in order to strengthen the case for admission to a sceptical Registrar.'[74]

When it was announced that Bethnal Green Hospital was to be closed, Widgery did not clap his hands. He believed the area could ill afford to lose such a valuable service, stating that the decision 'takes no account of social deprivation or incidence of disease in awarding resources, relying simply on out-of-date mortality rates. The result is a geographical interpretation rather than a class one, generating the lunacy of designating areas like Tower Hamlets, Hackney and Brent as possessing more than their fair share of resources, which are therefore deemed suitable for siphoning off to East Anglia.'[75]

Widgery was elected Chair of the Save Bethnal Green Campaign. Petitions, podiums and protest marches were coordinated. His experience in grass-roots activism meant that he was able to draw support from other industries. Despite popular support, they failed to provoke the desired government response. When things were getting desperate and closure looked imminent, a casualty work-in began. Staff occupied the building and continued to treat patients, going against government wishes to see it shut. This was an operation that required everyone, from cleaner to consultant, to be involved. Widgery described the event.

> On July 1978, after a ten-month campaign to keep Bethnal Green Hospital open, the first-ever casualty work-in began. The run-up to the work-in had included one of the largest post-war political meetings ever held in the York Hall, the famous boxing venue, a petition signed by 20 000 people and a thirteen-point objection signed by 102 East-End GPs, a march of 500 people in wheelchairs and bandages and a two-hour protest strike from which workers from all five local hospitals were joined by brewery workers, printers, postal workers and strikers from other industries.[76]

These tactics generated much-needed media attention. *News at Ten* would hardly have rolled out the cameras to film the signing of a petition. Such pressure was compounded by union support. The day after the work-in began, the National Union of Public Employees voted in favour of 'immediate industrial action in the case of any attempt to close the Casualty Department at Bethnal Green'.[77] A representative from the Department of Health finally agreed to meet the campaigners, but the government was not prepared to change its position. Two weeks later Bethnal Green was closed forever. During the course of the work-in, which lasted 30 days, 1100 emergency patients were treated.[77]

In some ways it was remarkable that such a campaign started in the first place. We need to remember how isolated Widgery felt during the early 1970s. The notion of unified industrial action, with little dialogue between the hospital factions, was to him whimsical. By the end of the 1970s everyone in the NHS was threatening strikes. (There was a slight irony in this for Widgery; direct action by consultants prevented the removal of private pay-beds from NHS hospitals.) But despite the failure of the Bethnal Green work-in, we see – if we squint our eyes ever so slightly – that it succeeded in other ways.

If the hospital had closed without protest, there would have been no story for national television. The campaign made ordinary people, not simply those making the decision, aware of what was going on. This was not an isolated event; other hospitals had already been threatened and more were to follow. The Bethnal Green campaign encouraged others, like the one to save the Elizabeth Garrett Anderson Hospital (EGA), in what socialists might describe as 'perpetual revolution'. Having threatened the EGA with closure in 1976, in 1979 the Conservative government overturned the decision. Not least, Bethnal Green also provided many with an introduction to socialist politics.

The cuts, which started in the 1970s, continued long into the 1980s and beyond. The extent of the hospital closures is summed up by Widgery in *Limehouse Doctor*: 'When I first came here, there were 14 hospitals, now there's only three left.'

There were some people who felt that Widgery was slightly naive in his approach. Turner states that the hospitals were often small and poorly run without any overall coherence. 'In terms of the practical ability to deliver A&E care, it was the only viable solution. I was in favour of these closures because my perspective (working as a night chemist to pay medical fees) was these were small units that were badly run. Instead of having one coherent unit you had half a dozen all doing different things.'

Turner points out that the closures represented a cut for only very local people, those who used Accident and Emergency instead of a GP.[*] 'Part of Dave's fury about defending every small crappy outpost of the NHS was because in fact he hadn't done a lot of practical medicine at that time. When I first met Dave [in the late 1970s] he'd just started working at a regular practice three days a week, alongside his writing. He was getting down to the basics of what it was like delivering healthcare to an East-End population.'

Widgery did not have blind love for the hospitals. Following the closure of Poplar Hospital in 1974 Widgery wrote, 'Nobody, least of all the patients and staff of the threatened hospitals in East London, or the many

---

[*] The closure of hospitals came during a time when most GPs were single-handed practices. Health centres were only starting up.

other parts of Britain where the same battles are in the offing, are arguing that these old hospitals are the answer. However hard you try to overcome it, they are grim and still bear the stamp of the Poor Law. If health care really was developing in Britain, these hospitals would probably be best developed as local community hospitals, run mainly by GPs, and housing day centres for the old, nurseries and antenatal and childcare centres which fitted what is needed for the continuous good health of the working class and not the emergencies of accidents and acute illness.'[78]

Turner accepts that the East End got a raw deal. 'What's interesting is that there are many nicer hospitals in the West End than the East End.' He believes that the new building for the Chelsea and Westminster, which ran £50 million over budget, was the reason why Homerton Hospital took so long to be moved from its previously destitute site. The money promised to Homerton was £50 million.

Widgery applied the tactics of direct action. In the same way he had tried to convert the community in Chapel Market as a young member of IS, he strove to convert those communities whose hospitals were being threatened. The socialist idea behind this was that you encouraged workers to take control of their own conditions of employment, not to be reliant on managers. Medicine, in terms of Widgery's global socialist vision, was just part of the picture.

Stethoscope, telephone, dictaphone, prescription pad, local medical meetings, petitions, marches, podiums, hospital occupations – these were the armaments with which Widgery fought for his ideals as a medical practitioner. Despite such an extensive list, we are in danger of overlooking his most powerful weapon of all.

Chapter 6

Written words prescribed

We are surprised if the doctor, by stealing some hours from his daily avocations, attains even moderate eminence in the path of literature.[79]

Edward Berdoe

You advise me not to pursue two hares at a time and to abandon the practice of medicine ... I feel more contented and more satisfied when I realise that I have two professions, not one. Medicine is my lawful wife and literature my mistress: when I grow weary of one, I pass the night with the other. This may seem disorderly, but it is not dull, and besides, neither of them suffers because of my infidelity. If I did not have my medical work, it would be hard to give my thought and liberty to literature.[80]

Anton Chekhov

Part of Widgery's appeal is that he wrote. He did not give up the arts in a world of science. Sometimes it is reassuring to hear that people have been able to pursue outside interests. Not just for those who are not yet qualified, but for those who feel caught up in the thick of things. It confirms that you can get off the motorway from time to time. Some will say that this detracts from the important commitment needed for medicine. An argument could be made, however, that outside interests feed back into medicine, making for better doctors. As Rhona MacDonald, who edits the *BMJ* careers section argues, 'There are many doctors who still love medicine and are satisfied with their careers. They often have outside interests as well, such as writing children's books, being a stand-up comic, and running an art gallery. Could this be the answer to fulfilment, happiness and therefore "goodness"? I wonder.'[81]

Bertrand Russell certainly seemed to share the view that a diverse and multifaceted life was a good thing. In 1935 he wrote an essay entitled 'In praise of idleness', an argument for working only four hours a day. It is a wonderful notion that with 'a certain very moderate amount of sensible organisation' everyone would have a job and the material needs of the population would be met.[82] This is not the only reason why the four-hour day would be good. Russell believes it represents a window of opportunity, which he describes in the following extract with just a smidgeon of gender bias. It was, after all, the 1930s.

> In a world where no one is compelled to work more than four hours a day, every person possessed of scientific curiosity will be able to indulge it, and every painter will be able to paint without starving, however excellent his pictures may be. Young writers will not be obliged to draw attention to themselves by sensational pot-boilers, with a view to acquiring the economic independence needed for monumental works, for which, when the time at last comes, they will have lost the taste and the capacity. Men who, in their professional work, have become interested in some phase of economics or government, will be able to develop their ideas without the academic detachment that makes the work of university economists seem lacking in reality. Medical men will have time to learn about the progress of medicine.[83]

While literature symbolises 'idleness' in the sense described above, it actually occupies a particularly close relationship with medicine. This is apparent in two ways: reading creative writing, and the act of writing itself. John Salinsky, himself a GP in Wembley, believes that an interest in literature helps him to understand his patients' feelings better and, in doing so, to become less frustrated with them. 'If you were to call all this an enhanced capacity for empathy, I should not disagree … I would certainly maintain that a writer like Tolstoy (when he is writing fiction) can tell you more about what it is to be human and have feelings than any number of textbooks of psychology or handbooks of psychotherapy.'[84]

Medicine has produced its fair share of landmark authors. Keats, Chekhov and Conan Doyle (to name but a few) were all doctors. Dr Russell Brain, the President of the Royal College of Physicians, strove to articulate this special relationship. Writing in 1952 he stated, 'The doctor occupies a seat in the front row of the stalls of the human drama, and is constantly watching, and even intervening in, the tragedies, comedies and tragic comedies which form the raw material of the literary art. If the doctor is capable of his work, he must be a man of feeling; and if he is to do his work, feelings must often in great measure be denied expression.'[85] In other words, doctors, who hold so much back, are filled with emotions waiting to explode. On the other hand, we could argue that this is nonsense. Such doctors would be writing regardless of whether or not they practised medicine.

Writing allowed David Widgery to touch people far beyond the consulting room. It provided the ultimate platform to reflect on the world and provoke thought in others. Widgery admits he was inspired by William Carlos Williams, an American GP who was awarded the Pulitzer Prize for Literature in 1963. For many people, Widgery was a writer first and a GP only later. Starting off with a sexually explicit school magazine, he ended up with a regular column in the *BMJ*. It is to his development as a writer and his use of writing as a weapon that we now turn.

Origins of the writing

> Dave wanted to make people well. He felt for the fact that people were suffering in all these bloody horrible places. But his most effective weapon for doing that was as a polemicist, as a writer, and as a bloke appearing on the television screen. David was God's gift to all these things ... He'd flick his large eyes at the camera and everyone would say 'Christ, yes!' That is a great virtue.
>
> Nigel Fountain

Widgery's passion for writing can be found in his youth. Reading was one of the few forms of escapism permitted to a polio sufferer. In his enforced isolation, the ideas that shaped his outlook on the world were found and cherished. Speaking to Tony Gould for the book *A Summer Plague: polio and its survivors*, he said, 'I think the reason I became left wing was because I read a lot, and I read a lot because I had a lot of time on my hands. I was converted to left-wing ideals by reading Bertrand Russell and Bernard Shaw and people like that, and I think probably my mother's influence – she was a left-wing Methodist verging on Quakerism, which was about as far left as you could go in the Thames Valley in those days.'[86]

This childhood pursuit became an integral part of his existence. He read at a fantastic rate throughout his life. Michael Rosen, the broadcaster and children's author, would always be amazed by the volume of material Dave 'The Doctor' read. They were keen literary friends and published a collection of their favourite subversive prose in the *Chatto Book of Discontent*. Widgery would often badger him for an opinion about the book he had just read. Michael would reply, 'Christ, Dave, I've got to have time to write as well!'

One of Widgery's major inspirational literary events was the discovery of Jack Kerouac's *On The Road*. 'To read Kerouac when you were 15, scribbling through the Ks of Slough Public Library, was a coded message of discontent; the sudden realisation of an utter subversivness and licence.' For Widgery it legitimised experimentation with the written word. No longer did strict rules apply. The colours of the palette had merged and the possibilities were infinite. 'I, like ten thousand other fifth formers, wrote a series of letters in imitation of Kerouac, spiralling indiscriminate word patterns and being able, in his shadow, to write thewordstogether if I so wanted.'

Widgery loved artists who had gone out and achieved something new: the Romantics – Rimbaud, Shelley and Keats; people who had pushed back the boundaries of experience, and in doing so produced work that strove to capture the universe. He was also a great admirer of the American poet Alan Ginsberg. A review of Ginsberg's work reflects elements that inspired Widgery's creative outlook on the world. 'In his North American romantic agony Ginsberg quite literally put himself through the extremes of drug experimentation, sexual iconoclasm, incessant travel and insanity to find and formulate his own visions of human possibility.'

There are, in fact, great similarities between the view that Widgery had of Ginsberg and the view others had of Widgery. As Michael Rosen put it, 'Whatever he was doing he was pushing himself to the very extreme. He once tried to explain to me that form of extremism about pushing our body and mind to limit. However, it was like trying to talk to a Tory about peace ... "You have one life therefore you should try everything. Go for all the extremes. This society keeps trying to narrow your options."'[13]

Widgery wrote about anything and everything. As a journalist, historian, letter writer, book reviewer and political author, the expanse of his subject interest was vast. His writings spanned art, France, music, theatre, books, politics, health and many more topics. His passions and interests were his writings. When something grabbed his attention, like what you were saying in a conversation, he would write it down. This earned him the reputation, amongst his friends, of a literary magpie. Other people's lines would disappear to reappear in print. He was never too proud to steal someone else's words.

During his life he wrote for various publications. Articles appeared in political publications like *City Limits, Oz, Rank and File Teacher, Socialist Review, Temporary Hoarding, Time Out* (which was known for 'espousing libertarian and authoritarian politics'[87] before changing management to become the publication London knows today), *Socialist Worker, Radical America*. He also contributed to more mainstream publications like *New Society, The Guardian, The Observer, The Independent on Sunday*, and not forgetting the *BMJ*. One piece of writing seems to fall outside this category. Much to the amusement of his friends, during his *Oz* heyday, he was commissioned to write an article for *Playboy* for a feature on the British aristocracy.

Reading Widgery's work it is easy to appreciate his talent. He captivated his readers, whisking them along with witty poetic imagery. This is demonstrated in the following extract from an article he wrote about Canary Wharf.

I first came to the East End over twenty years ago and it still seems like only yesterday; the loveliness of the ships at night on the still water behind the high dock walls; the public bars full of sailors, dockers and artists flooded with beer and brilliantine; the deep pungent precipices formed by the warehouses. The Isle of Dogs was still self-enclosed in psychology and maritime in spirit; and the Cockney was a specifically East-End argot. . . . There was jazz as well as jobs and you didn't have to get out of the borough when you grew up. There seemed to be places to court, to cry, to quarrel and make up, to grow old with grace and children still in reach.[88]

Imagery and description were always cemented by strong opinions. In the same article he writes, 'What is most striking about this vast commercial folly is not the pretensions of the architecture, sort of Croydon-on-Thames pretending to be Chicago, but the lack of people . . . the free market metropolis has replaced genuine *quartiers populaires* with spaces designed to exclude ordinary people . . . We needed mixed use of land, low-rent housing, smaller scale manufacturing, informal places. Instead we got the future according to (government funded) estate agents. And it doesn't work.'

Widgery was never one to shy away from being offensive. Roland Muldoon remembers a letter Widgery wrote, attacking a campaign for democracy in Rhodesia that CAST were part of during the early 1970s. They had organised a benefit gig called 'Psycadelfia vs. Ian Smith'. Muldoon confesses, 'We were going to give the money to buy guns for the revolution.' Part of the campaign meant collaborating with an existing group of people who had started selling car stickers, which read 'Rhodesia: One Man One Vote'. Widgery's letter was the first encounter between the two men. Despite the friendship that ensued in later years, Muldoon is still annoyed. 'Widgery wrote a stinging letter in the *New Statesman* saying what white middle-class fuck-wits we must be. "One man, one vote. Not socialism, not changing the world; creepy crappy reformism." It really pissed us off. He implied that we were all City workers, while I at the time was working on the Victoria Line, on the underground. He just assumed that we were Hampstead-ites.'[46]

Widgery created time for writing when you would expect other pressures to prevail. For example, in his retrospective collection of his work, *Preserving Disorder*, he stated that, 'During the 1970s . . . I was working as a doctor in acute hospital medicine while attempting to write while on call or early in the morning.'[89]

There was something about him that wanted to document everything, to preserve it. History was slipping away with every second. Tony Benn,[*]

---

[*] Tony Benn was a Labour parliamentarian of fifty years who retired in 2000. He is famous for his socialist views and his published diaries.

who records political events in his diary and with his handheld video camera, has a similar attribute: the need to preserve events for future generations, something especially important to both socialists. They hold true to a certain interpretation of history, believing that past events provide strong evidence for future change.

Writing at such a furious pace, in an already compact life, had consequences. Ian Birchall recalled 'a man who was moving so quickly that he never bothered to correct his mistakes. All his books are brilliant, and they're all riddled with inaccuracies. If you write like that, in his sort of way, then checking the spelling of Leighton Buzzard isn't the most important thing.'[90] Sheila Rowbotham, from a historian's perspective, would often find her jaw dropping. 'The historian's guilt at inaccuracy was merely bizarre to him.'[91] Paul Foot, former editor of *Socialist Worker*, admits that such haphazardness was compensated by a streak of brilliance. 'At times, lying in bed at night with the *Socialist Worker* pages rolling around in the darkness, I would yearn for some plain good prose, something which people would enjoy reading for its own sake, even if the line was slightly dubious. There were so few who wrote like that: Peter Sedgwick did, so did Eamon McCann; and so, always, did David Widgery.'[90]

David Renton, in his essay 'The poetics of propaganda', argues that Widgery was as good a political writer as George Orwell. He makes the comparison between Orwell's six rules for avoiding bad political writing, taken from *Politics and the English Language*, and Widgery's own prose. 'Like Orwell, Widgery wrote in a style that treasured originality and creativity. He was aware that communication took place through the reader's imagination and not just through passive acceptance of the printed word. His writing style played with styles and images to create meaning. It was a very simple musical language.' Renton continues to suggest that from Widgery political writers can take away two more rules: first, 'Always write for your audience'; and second, 'Don't just write for your audience, challenge them.'

For Widgery, writing was like moaning over a pint of beer after a stressful day. Albeit with an important difference. It was about changing things. As Juliet Ash explained, 'He saw writing as a viable tool to get ideas across in terms of communicating to people. Such people are then able to take these ideas and use them to effectively counter government policy. For him writing was something that he could do instantly. I don't think he ever felt that he would never be able to have a part, or a voice, against government.'[92] He often wrote impulsively. If there were things annoying him, 'he would either rage or write. He would often come home and write a quick letter to *The Guardian*.'[92] Many of his articles, drawing heavily on his medical experience, were not intended for a medical readership. He was always angling for a wider audience. 'Blood on the lino: 24 hours in Casualty', published in *Time Out* in 1976, is a typical example. Working as a casualty officer in Bethnal Green Hospital, Widgery was keen to bring home to people the reality he knew. 'The world of Casualty is like a gravity-less lunar capsule where limbs and surfaces are continually colliding and objects constantly tumble and drop.' He is soon voicing his frustration. 'The job is exhausting, bewildering and, since it places paramount importance on diagnosis and little on treatment, curiously unsatisfactory. Shift work, low pay and lower prestige, generally poor facilities and lack of career structure has made Casualty a dead end.'

What initially appears like a personally motivated piece about working conditions, in a discipline that at the time was without much of a career structure, soon turns into a hard-hitting reflection about problems infecting his community. He argues against those who hold up the 'sanctity of the family as a solution to all our problems'. He challenges them to 'spend a few hours in Casualty, to face the debris, when all the sugary ideals explode, when babies are bounced against the bedroom wall to make them stop crying and wives are loved and honoured and beaten up so thoroughly that they can't talk because their teeth are still chattering with terror'.[89]

It was Widgery's overriding ambition, according to many of his friends, to become a writer. We have seen how at medical school he eloped into the underground press. He was forever scribbling. Even when he became a doctor, he still worked through the night to publish another issue of *Temporary Hoarding*. But at some point Widgery changed; his desire to become a writer subsided, his passion for general practice increased. As we heard from Ruth Gregory earlier, this was partly because he held an over-romantic belief in what it was to be a writer. Writing, he found, was not going to pay his bills. At the same time, he became genuinely fired by what he saw as a doctor. The twist is that by the late 1980s these seemingly separate passions, medicine and writing, were entwined. Their interaction allowed him to write two books about healthcare and to get a column in the *BMJ*.

The National Health

The National Health, A Radical Perspective was published in 1988 as an updated version of *Health in Danger* (1978). Published by Pluto Press, it provides a historical account of healthcare in Britain, with particular emphasis on the trials and tribulations of the NHS. It is worth mentioning something about the period in which it was written.

Since taking power in 1979, the Conservative government had sought to increase competition within the NHS, believing it would increase efficiency. Despite claims that more money was going into the NHS, by the mid-1980s, leaders of the profession remained unhappy.[93] In London, cuts of £35 million from district budgets, and the closure of 2500 acute beds, were affecting service and morale. It was against this backdrop that the book was published. Widgery confesses in the introduction that it was written 'sometimes in anger, sometimes in sorrow, in the gaps between my full-time work as an East London GP. It is an attempt to unravel just what is happening to our Health Service and to explain the implications to the public who rely on it. It is also an attempt to restate the socialist case for comprehensive and democratic health care. And in the process it is an attack on the public spending cuts which, in the late eighties, threaten the existence of the NHS.'

The book is a radically eclectic history of healthcare in Britain. Its main focus is the NHS. Nevertheless, Widgery takes time to explain what health provision was like before the NHS began. It is a class-based analysis intended to demonstrate how far healthcare had progressed. 'The rich endured their treatment in their homes, selecting their physicians from the Royal Colleges on the basis of snobbery, nepotism or their man's reputation in the voluntary hospitals, where aspiring doctors quite literally practised on the poor.'[94]

Widgery challenges the perception that the formation of the NHS was inevitable. He reminds us of the many professional interests that were at stake. GPs wanted to remain in control of their own working conditions. Consultants wanted to protect the high earnings they had enjoyed before, which essentially meant preserving the right to private practice. Widgery points out that the end product was a result of interplay between noble intentions and interested parties. 'Although Nye Bevan* had a keen appreciation of the limitations of his reforms within the existing social framework, he was unable and politically unwilling to challenge them. He sought to exact the best possible compromise within the existing balance of power by gaining the support of the most influential section of the medical world, the consultants and the Royal Colleges, by "stuffing their mouths with gold".'

Widgery reflects the sentiment shared by the Socialist Health Association. When plans were being drawn up for the NHS they argued that while it was good, it was not good enough. This line of thought remains consistent throughout the book. In a chapter on 'The drugs industry', Widgery questions the role of pharmaceutical companies and their relationship with the NHS. He appears sceptical as to whether their inter-

---

* Bevan was responsible for drawing up plans for the NHS in post-war Britain.

ests are compatible. 'It is ironic that the industry with the most honourable of purposes, the relief of suffering, exhibits the most piratical features of modern big business ... The drug companies' influence is no longer merely financial. They do much to mould research, therapy, education and the whole ethos of contemporary medicine ... Put simply, there are now too many drugs produced. They are overpriced and misleadingly promoted. Their overconsumption is itself a cause of illness, their over-prescription a substitute for clinical skill, and their overpricing a crucial cause of the poverty of the NHS.'[95]

If you thought the employment structure within the NHS exemplified egalitarian multiculturalism, *The National Health* makes us think again. Widgery describes it as a 'pyramid of power with the wealthy, white, male consultant at its pinnacle and the Asian and Caribbean women cleaners, cooks and ward nurses toiling away, underpaid and under-appreciated, at the base'.[96] His words resound with controversy encouraging the reader to think. Do teaching hospitals really, as Widgery claims, 'produce a medical profession out of touch with reality; geographically located in the inner city, ideologically located in the Home Counties'?[97]

What could be interpreted as a barrage of criticism is countered by a belief that change is possible. People need to disagree, to stand up when they could easily not. 'In this imperfect and worsening world we desper-ately need our doctors, our hospitals, our nurses and our ancillaries. We need them to be given finances to use their skill to the full. The cuts must be stopped and spending increased to a level at which the NHS can func-tion properly again. Until this is done, we – health workers, patients and citizens – must raise our level of dissent.' Widgery reminds us that bene-ficial changes in healthcare have not come about instantaneously, as if by magic. To illustrate this point he cites the case of Wendy Savage, the obste-trician suspended from her post during the 1980s. Colleagues at the Royal London Hospital alleged that she was incompetent. Supporters of her progressive approach thought this was slander by protectors of the old school. As Widgery explains, they believed it was a case of the 'high-tech, interventionist school of conventional obstetric care' trying to dismiss Savage's 'woman-centred, community-based approach'.[98]

A public enquiry subsequently reinstated her. Wendy Savage is now seen as something of a pioneer. The book reminds us that it could have been a very different story. 'If the enquiry had not been made public; if Mrs Savage had been represented by her original defence union-assigned solicitors; if her supporters had not taken her case to the streets, pubs, and markets of East London and to the media; if doctors in primary care, in contrast to the deafening silence from her hospital colleagues, had not backed her clinically, then the original attempt might have succeeded, dealing a serious blow to progressive obstetrics.'[99]

The overriding message behind the book, although not always that clear, is to 'convince more people that the health service is something worth fighting for. And that, in fighting for it, we may glimpse our ability to create a society run on a different and better basis.'[100] Socialism and good healthcare are in Widgery's eyes synonymous. While he believes there are problems within the NHS, the greatest problem exists outside. 'Most of all it has had to exist in a society whose central economic tenets are diametrically opposed to the values the NHS attempts to promulgate.'[101]

At a time when the link between poverty and ill health was very much ignored, Widgery had no doubt. 'It is my conviction that in a better society, no longer class-divided and profit driven, many of the medical problems now present would not exist. I like to think that there might even be a lot fewer doctors, social workers and do-gooders because good would be done by itself.'[102]

National reception

Widgery's ability to bring home the bleak reality of health policy is beyond question. One reviewer wrote, 'After reading the book, I was overwhelmed by feelings of gloom and despair.'[103] *The Observer*, in a review about books on the health service published around the same time, writes 'Widgery gives the clearest picture of the misery that cuts in the NHS are now causing.'[104] One of the main criticisms is that he perhaps attempts too much: 'The flair and even excitement of his writing cannot compensate for his lack of direction: his book covers too many topics and suggests no new strategy.'[104] This is a fair point. Widgery seems to have attempted to disclose every possible issue. The chapters are all interesting but they do not necessarily link. At the same time this is probably what led *Socialist Worker Review* to write, 'For anyone trying to fight the cuts or concerned about the future of the NHS, Widgery's book is an invaluable source of information.'[105]

The National Health is at times slapdash, perhaps a hallmark of Widgery's great speed. As a review in the *Journal of Advanced Nursing* complains, 'the cavalier approach to referencing is unforgivable, half the authors cited do not appear in the index, and the selection of end notes is partial'.[106] There are also moments in the text where Widgery is not totally honest. In describing the hospital closures and the campaign to save Bethnal Green, he writes, 'For as the Chairman of the Campaign wrote prophetically in 1980 ... "If we have awoken the general public to the seriousness of what lies ahead for the London NHS, we will have achieved something of real importance. It is better to have fought and won a partial victory than never to have stirred at all.'''[107] Widgery fails to explain that this quote is his own.

It is worth pointing out, with a slight deviation, that self-promotion was almost signature Widgery – often accompanied by distortion of the facts. One such example, appearing in his book *Temporary Hoarding*, is the use of a photograph taken during the 1967 'Battle for Grosvenor Square'. In the picture there appear a group of people carrying an injured protestor to safety. A youthful Nigel Fountain and David Widgery are in the foreground, their arms locked around the legs of the victim of police brutality. Fountain, with more hair than he possesses today, is bleeding on the right side of his face. Widgery, with a rather large fur collar to his leather jacket, looks open-mouthed and earnestly off-camera. The caption reads, without identifying the people, 'Student Revolutionaries storm the American Embassy'.[108] Over 20 years later Fountain tells a less revolutionary tale. He was bleeding because he fell whilst running towards the embassy. He got the bruise from falling off Widgery's motorbike a few days prior. 'This was very useful because it meant I could sit down and be tended, whilst David could sit around being a doctor.' Let us return to the medical world.

With *The National Health* there is a feeling that Widgery lacks solutions to the problems he articulates. 'He never develops beyond a stance which sees the Labour Movement as the only really important actor. He ends

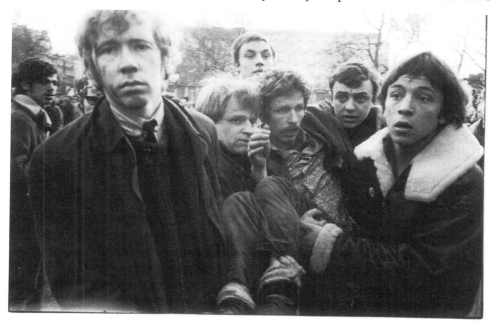

Student revolutionaries storm the American Embassy. Nigel Fountain in left foreground, David Widgery on right. Photographer unknown.

with a call for more money and more militancy. All this is not enough.'[109] Widgery argues that healthcare can be improved in two ways. First, those concerned with the progress of the health service are, like football fans, entitled to make demands. Dissent on the terraces needs to be increased. Government will in turn listen to these voices. There is nothing wrong with such claims, but it is worth remembering that by 1988 the Labour Movement was no longer as powerful as it had once been.

Second, Widgery alludes to a more global solution. He talks of a world where doctors are no longer needed, where society heals itself. Explicit instructions about how this world can be achieved are lacking. This is frustrating. Such a problem was something that preoccupied many Marxist groups. As Fountain wondered, 'How does the Marxist party live in a capitalist world, offering solutions within that world which may lead onto something else? ... That was never David's strong point. He was wonderful for leaps of imagination, falling about laughing, explaining the absurdity of the system. When he applied that great brain of his to unsentimental description and polemicism, he was wonderful.'[20]

In Widgery's defence, he articulates something similar during the early 1990s, but appears to have a more mature perspective. 'In a society that was organised on a different basis, which took human needs as its starting point, a society without this insane competition which produces so much unhappiness in the pursuit of so called happiness ... I think there would be a lot less ill health. And the ill health that there was, would be dealt with much better but that really would be talking about a very very different society. It is difficult to imagine how we, in our society, would get there but that's what matters ... how we go from where we are now to this other place.'[49]

Passionate polemics is what Widgery did best, prompting leading commentator Professor Rudolph Klein, having read *The National Health*, to write, 'The NHS needs people with the kind of humane idealism displayed by Dr Widgery.' For these very reasons his second book about healthcare is generally considered his best.

Some Lives!

In 1991 *Some Lives!: A GP's East End* was published by Sinclair Stevenson. The book, as Michael Rosen describes it, 'is a marriage of a sober historical analysis with a kind of impressionistic writing that actually owes its origins to his interest in psychedelic writing. The book is heartsy, gutsy ... It combines Dave's face-to-face encounters with patients with a historic account of the East End. It's unique. No one else could have done it.' It was a book that Widgery had always wanted to write.

The East End community Widgery served changed visibly during the 1980s. Big business moved in whilst local people were forced out. Such changes occurred in the wider context of further cuts within the health service. Widgery was saddened by these events. Underlying the text is his unstinting love for the East End, for an era which has passed. Recalling the East End of the 1950s and early 1960s [one that he never saw] he writes with a sense of romantic nostalgia, 'It may have had street prostitutes and red light districts, but little rape or child abuse was reported. There were buckets of beer but no heroin, set-piece gang battles but few random muggings.'[109] Hope, morale, and optimism have gone . . . I'm watching something die and I wish I wasn't. Perhaps the best I can do is record the process.'[110]

The book dwells on the changes in industry, housing and population the area had undergone, all of which affected Widgery's patients. 'The ship repair yards like Green and Silley Weir and Badgers closed in the mid-1970s. And the riverside food-processing, confectionery and biscuit manufacturers followed suit . . . the rate of growth in unemployment accelerated during the recession of the 1980s.'[111]

Developments like Canary Wharf failed to improve things during this period, making life tough for many people. 'Among one's patients, especially the over-fifties and the chronically sick, unemployment is a way of life, and I have with time had to alter the question "What is your job?" to "When did you last work?"'[109] Throughout the book he combines history and social commentary with personal anecdotes. *The Observer* wrote, 'This mixture of medicine and militancy makes for invigorating prose. The book is full of pungent asides on the urban condition, and it bristles with judgment too . . . '

We obtain a strong sense of how much Widgery loved the working-class people of the East End. 'How well the modern Cockneys do in circumstances their "betters" would find impossible. How much better they would do if their material conditions were hoisted a few notches up the class system. And yet how much more common decency, respect for humanity, honour and humour they possess than so many of the middle and upper classes who despite lip service to collective values in fact approach life in a spirit of naked self-interest.'[112]

There are some who would describe such a view as provocative (and perhaps slightly naive). The working classes are the heroes, the middle classes spoilt. 'The middle-class new birth visit is also to a slightly different world. The baby is still centre stage and the delight and pride are common. But the baby will already be clad in gender-non-specific primary colours and its first toy will be non-sweetening, design award-winning, psychologically appropriate mobiles rather than the pink or blue cuddly toys which arrive in the crib of the proletarian newborn.'[113] It is as though a person's class defines them automatically as a good or a bad person.

Widgery was obviously shocked by the levels of deprivation he saw, but, at the same time, he was inspired by the resilience he witnessed. From a community that people were ready to dismiss as doomed, Widgery is quick to highlight those aspects which he believes are positive. The impression is that working there can be an enriching and fascinating experience, like the diversity of people (from all over the world) who make up the East-End population.

Widgery highlights the many groups – Huguenots, Irish, East European Jews – who all settled in the East End, seeking escape from persecution, before the 20th century had even begun. Such writing takes on a greater meaning in the context of Widgery's previous work with RAR, where he was actively trying to disperse rising racist and violent sentiment. Immigration is not a new phenomenon. 'Contrary to popular belief, Asians have been seen in the East End for a long time, because the East India Company, whose monopoly was established in 1600, had its administrative headquarters in Poplar and the City.'[114]

Widgery points out that the above groups have had to struggle and endure hardship; all have proved that they have something valuable to contribute to the community. He cites the Jubilee Street Anarchist Club formed in 1906. This club was 'irreligious and for sexual equality ... above all it was a place where Shaw was listened to by tailors and shoe- and cabinet-makers hungry for ideas'.[115] All this giving credence to a struggle Widgery wants to protect.

In *Some Lives!* there is no substitute for experience. Its superficially apparent social-historical narrative is injected with life through personal anecdotes and extracts from Widgery's consultations. His stream of consciousness plunges in and out of pools of human experience. GPs are extremely well positioned to appreciate such diverse and rich insights. The text is an intriguing scrapbook. In order to convey its essence extensive quotation is required. We will start with a postnatal problem and follow him through a series of moments.

Disaster rides shotgun in the happy family, you've already been warned. Then a postnatal infection. Cluster of needle-headed boils on the perineum. But more importantly, Ruth Baxter is attempting to execute her baby: full-scale puerperal psychosis. 'When it rears its ugly head it goes straight to my stomach,' she says as I examine. When her husband's not looking she tries to throw the baby out of the window. Like Punch and Judy. Puerperal psychosis: 'a psychiatric emergency'. But so are all of them; cramped flats, every inch of space occupied, beds a battlefield, stairs lethal. Calls for drinks, calls for food, clothes to be found, children to be silenced, arguments about plans. Nobody agrees. Dad shouts. Mum cries. The children go silent. Ruth is florid. So she gets ECT.

'I want to choke them and poison them and shake them to pieces,' Mrs Svensen says.

'No jobs!' Svensen shouts. 'I was made redundant, wasn't I!'

'It's his stomach, you know,' says Mrs Svensen. Pause, meaningful. 'It aggravates. He was aggravated by the inspector. Business is slack so they'll use the least excuse. People will give a lot for a job these days.'

'Mustn't grumble,' says Svensen. 'Only got mugged, didn't I. Beer with friends, money stole, didn't see his face. They grab hold of things. We don't have the right to be considered. But my stamps are in order.'

Mrs Veitch, a strong woman, folds hands by sink. 'You'd better go and look at him.' He is tucked up in a bed like a wedge of cheese. A railway porter at Liverpool Street with a far-away look in his eyes. Once he told me, 'We're the working class and we'll never alter.' He has a darting toothy grin.

His death came on Good Friday in a room full of boxing photos. I was there. He said just before he died, 'You've been a good wife.' She said, 'Let's not talk like that.' She says afterwards, 'He went quiet. But he was big, I did my back in lifting him.'

She has a letter from her son:

'Dear Mum, I hope you are well and happy. Thank you for your letter. I was glad to hear that you got home alright even though you did go the long way round. I got a letter from Bill and he sent me £5 to buy papers. He said he was glad to hear I only got four years. I'm growing a beard because I'm fed up with shaving all the time but have come out in a rash. Prison isn't so bad. Sorry to hear about Dad.'[116]

WE WANT MORE MONEY FOR THE NHS BUT TO RAISE IT BY INCREASING PRESCRIPTION CHARGES IS TO PUT A TAX ON THE SICK WHO CAN LEAST AFFORD IT. IT IS TO TURN PHARMACISTS INTO TAX COLLECTORS AND MAKE DOCTORS THINK FIRST ABOUT THE PATIENT'S FINANCIAL STATE, RATHER THAN THE BEST AVAILABLE TREATMENTS.

If you agree with this leaflet please display it and distribute it.

The picture painted is rather grim. 'When I came here in that fateful taxi down the Hackney Road, I didn't know what the bruised face of a raped heroin addict was like, or how children could be locked up without food, four in a room, by a drunken father as a punishment, or what happens to a jaw when it is broken in a domestic fight and concealed. And now I do ... I think I wish I didn't.'

It is difficult to read about the conditions endured by the East-Enders without feeling shocked. You feel sorry for the patients and for the doctor. From these social ills sprout more problems, in what is seemingly a vicious circle.

Widgery tells us the social and personal cost of chronic unemployment, which 'breeds resentment and frustration which can all too easily be channelled into radicalism, xenophobia and chauvinism'.[117] Poverty leads to ill health and much more. He regards this as one of society's great injustices, refusing to accept that it is simply how the cards have been dealt. As he explains in the chapter 'Growing up tough', 'To believe that these inequalities are inevitable is to believe that the working class children somehow need less fresh air and fewer books and smaller bedrooms. That they are in some way less human than the children born elsewhere. And to accept that, especially if you are in a position to do something about it, would require a terrible cruelty.'[118]

As well as conveying a serious and sombre reflection on society, the journey through *Some Lives!* is eased by humour. This is arguably one of the most important pieces of equipment in any doctor's bag: the ability to make heavy circumstances light. Whilst describing his bus journey to work, Widgery writes, 'On the front of the bus is a London Transport poster which announces "Graffiti is Vandalism". I think it goes on to say "Vandalism is crime". But it has been vandalised'.[119]

Some lives received

Some Lives! made a large impact. Extracts and reviews were featured in many magazines and newspapers. The reviewers were full of praise. As Harriet Harman wrote in *The Independent on Sunday*, 'David Widgery doesn't need to lie awake pondering the meaning of life. He has found it in his daily work, fighting for patients whose life chances are whittled away before they are even born. He is a medical missionary who challenges not just the government but the values of society as a whole.'[120]

Some Lives! was described by *The Lancet* as 'a political book with a human heart which is a delight to read'. Steve Iliffe, writing in the *BMJ*, called it 'a Viennese pastry of a book' with Widgery's 'sharp ear, honest and accurate eye and a fine writing style making the book irresistible'.[121] The success of *Some Lives!* was fuelled further by the popularly perceived failure of Canary Wharf. A headline in *GP News* proclaimed: 'GP can say "I told you so" after Canary Wharf fails'. The article went on: 'Sales of his book, which forecast the collapse, soared when the developers admitted their insolvency last month.'[122] Widgery is quick to gloat about the situation, as the report explains, 'He says he has enjoyed the financial crisis facing the developers Olympia and York and a series of desperate manoeuvres to save the project. Dr Widgery said: I'm enjoying it everyday. It's replaced *Eastenders* as my main source of entertainment.'

The lack of solutions to the problems articulated is a reoccurring criticism, as voiced in the *BMJ* review. '*Some Lives!* is understandably soft on solutions for hard-pressed doctors in a beleaguered population, and ends with a disappointing cliché, a complaint about the loss of soul of the community.' But Iliffe is quick to suggest that the book is itself a cure for the author. 'By romanticising about an impoverished but diverse community he is able to maintain his affection and enthusiasm for it and continue to work hard and effectively with people who greatly need his help. This is perhaps as good a coping strategy as any, tailored as it is for any pugnacious personalities in dramatic environments. Whether it would work for less courageous or self-confident doctors in the heart of sink estates on the edges of other cities, where neither past nor present offers a shred of glamour, is another matter.'

Many people close to Widgery felt that he was greatly saddened by what he saw as a GP on a daily basis. The community of Limehouse was full of deep-rooted social problems that were not easily cured. It is not exactly full of glamour. But presumably Widgery would have found a spark in general practice wherever he was, as long as it was not too affluent an area. Inequalities were, he believed, a consequence of the capitalist economic system; he believed that the ills of society could be treated with socialism. This is idealistic but it is a different interest to that portrayed in *Some Lives!* – namely, a love for the community of the East End. Such a view of the situation would presumably help doctors with socialist ideals regardless of where they were practising, i.e. 'where neither past nor present offers a shred of glamour'.

It was Widgery's failure to mention class struggle that his friend Kambiz Boomla saw as an imperfection. 'There is no mention of how people can help themselves, e.g. community associations in council estates.' Unions and collective actions are mentioned only from a retrospective perspective: a force from the past that has come to pass. The book, unlike *The National Health*, does not finish by saying, 'Wake up! It's time for you to do something.' There are perhaps two reasons for this.

It is possible that by the 1990s Widgery had become downbeat about the efficacy of such organised resistance. Compared to the climate of 1968, optimism was in short supply. His previous description of the 'convergence of a dissident and political intelligentsia with a mass and rebellious youth movement'[123] combined with the advice to 'greet and welcome anarchy'[123] would have seemed inappropriate. Second, it is possible that his decision to omit an explicitly socialist directive was a calculated one. Widgery toned down his opinions to try to appeal to a more mainstream audience. Raging revolution might put readers off. Even so, *Some Lives!* is perhaps the first step towards a solution. If no problems are articulated, no solutions will be found. It is impossible to read *Some Lives!* without pondering what might be done to make a difference. Without it being spelt out for them, people might inevitably view redistribution of wealth as an obvious course of action.

Widgery's portrayal of the East End is rather polarised. The working classes are idolised and held up for all to admire. Their circumstances may be tough, but somehow, with a little dose of human spirit, they survive. So abysmal was the picture he painted, in fact, that Anna Livingstone recalls receiving a message of sympathy following the publication of an extract of *Some Lives!* Yet despite what the book depicts, not everyone in the East End had it so tough. Many people enjoyed a reasonable standard of living but presumably their lives were not as interesting to read about. Certainly they would detract from the correlation between deprivation and ill health Widgery is trying to stress. Nevertheless *Some Lives!* was believed by many to have been the crowning literary achievement of his career.

The *British Medical Journal*

By the 1990s Widgery was regularly contributing to the *BMJ*, the most prestigious and widely read medical periodical in the country. A newly appointed editor called Richard Smith invited Widgery to write one of the first opinion columns in the journal. Precious paragraphs provided him with an opportunity to reflect and comment on events in the medical world and beyond. It might seem strange that Widgery, with all his famously anti-establishment views, should end up writing for the house magazine of the medical profession. Richard Smith points out that Widgery's contributions were more than welcome. 'We were trying to make the journal more political. The *BMJ* had a tradition of being far more radical, lobbying government for changes, at the beginning of the 20th century. With our columnists we try and have a range of opinions, and we also require that they write to a standard that is above and beyond what we normally require from contributers. Widgery was an exceptional writer.'[124]

According to Juliet Ash, Widgery was extremely proud to be writing for such a publication. It presented a great chance to communicate his views of the world to a wider audience. Iona Heath reflects that, 'I don't think you can write in the *BMJ* without a lot of people becoming aware of you.'[125] Equally, his appointment fed into the side of Widgery that wanted wider recognition (a theme we shall be exploring in the next chapter).

His columns were a fusion of *Some Lives!* and *The National Health*. Entertaining anecdotes (both contemporary and historical) were combined with serious reflections on the NHS, society and government policy: 'I once looked after a patient who had his leg shot off by mistake, and was given a pub as a macabre consolation prize.'[126]

Widgery obviously enjoyed writing for his middle-class readership; though a slightly patronising tone perhaps comes creeping through, as if he has the upper hand of experience. In one article he complains at length about the theft of his car radio, although it transpires that he is not that annoyed – a local pirate radio station prevented him from receiving Radio Three long before his radio was stolen. Through his reflections on the everyday he challenges what he assumes, rightly or wrongly, the majority of his *BMJ* readers take for granted.

From the light and anecdotal comes the more profound and universal. This is what he does exceptionally well. In another of his articles, he starts off with a historical reflection about the Association of Poor Law Doctors. He imagines what this 19th-century factional medical group would have thought about today's healthcare. Widgery writes, 'They would have complained bitterly about the degree of social distress. And excoriated the indifference of the rest of the profession to their daily experience of the laissez faire social policy.' This anecdote is a clever stepping stone to the subject he really wants to talk about, a recent meeting of the Association of General Practices in Urban Deprived Areas (AGUDA). It becomes an article of compare and contrast. For a start there would have been few female doctors at the 19th-century meetings. Nevertheless there are similarities – 'the inadequacy of liberal social policy, the crisis in housing for the poor, the problems of intoxicant abuse, and the gulf that has now opened between the state's claims for its health services and the local reality'.

Widgery seems able to bring local realities to life, striking the chord of everyday recognition. He talks about the 1990 contract which had placed certain constraints on medical practice, like targets for childhood immunisations and cervical cytology. Government policy causes unnecessary interference: 'The new work generated and the new financial regime which went with it were simply distracting workers from the attempt to reverse the inverse care law and provide better quality primary care in the city.'

The word of the person in the front line is often more valuable than the rhetoric of the politician. They do not have an agenda as transparent as the politician who visits a health centre days before an election. And this is what Widgery implies. He makes it clear that the concerns voiced at the AGUDA meeting were 'not coming from medical politicians or even the medical warhorses of the LMC Conference but from the people who wield the speculums and give the jabs themselves', from 'the people who have time to attend the at-risk case conferences, sort out the methadone scripts, and patch up the victims of racial attack'.

Widgery did provoke debate with some of his opinion pieces. In 'Desert Storm' he wrote about the 1991 invasion of Iraq. 'Far from unlocking the longstanding problems of the region, the "success" of Desert Storm seems to have encouraged Israel, which remains in cheerful violation of many UN resolutions ... And back in the United States, Bush's warrior glamour looks distinctly strained as he flips flops on the problems facing most Americans.' Widgery attacks the arguments that the war was horrible but it had to be done. It received a stinging letter, 'Widgery and similar propagandists never offer a better line of action that leaders of Western democracies might have taken. How would he have dealt with Nazi Germany? ... Widgery should realise that the road to the concentration camp, like the road to hell, is paved with good intentions.'[127]

'The Prince and the Psychiatrists', a piece about Prince Charles' talk at the 150th anniversary of the Royal College of Psychiatrists also provoked criticism. Widgery wrote, 'The problem is not the prince but the professionals who nowadays seem to have convinced themselves that the only way to get back in touch with the voice of the common man is to invite the heir to the throne along.'[128] There were some who felt this was harsh because the prince was speaking out against stigma, something that is a real problem with mental illness. Most amusing is the background to Widgery writing this piece. Trevor Turner had invited Widgery along to speak at the meeting. Somehow the schedule got changed, so that Prince Charles could speak at the beginning of the occasion rather than the end. 'We all got shuffled off into this big hall to wait for Prince Charles. And Dave was so pissed off with this ... So he got up and tried to walk out. Unfortunately the door he chose was a broom cupboard. Then when he finally left, a few minutes later he ended back up in the main hall.' Widgery consequently had to listen to the talk given by Prince Charles.

Kambiz Boomla was of the impression that Widgery's column in the *BMJ* was undertaken light-heartedly. It was just journalism, something he enjoyed doing. Iona Heath, on the other hand, believed that his columns represented something more significant – an explicitly political tool. 'He wrote fantastic things in the *BMJ*. I think an awful lot of people knew of him. He would write in a polemic way. He always had this thing of expressing solidarity with patients, which is a fairly unusual way of writing. If you want to change things, you don't do it with tables and numbers. He had a great journalistic skill.'[125]

These differing views reflect the relationship the readers had with Widgery. Kambiz knew Widgery through the IS. The *BMJ* therefore probably seemed to him less politically charged than the underground press. On the other hand to Iona, who only knew of Widgery much later, these articles inevitably seemed fresh and progressive.

There is something especially fascinating about Widgery's ability to make impressions in different spheres of society. He possessed an ability to pick things up from places where they might be considered mundane and drop them into areas where they became fresh and exciting. Writing about political issues is going to sound familiar if you write for a political audience. If, however, you write about political issues for an audience who have not really heard the arguments, the writing becomes fresh. The same is true with his medical experiences. Writing for the *BMJ* was not simply writing for East-End GPs. People who faced similar predicaments to him up and down the country, who perceived similar inequalities, would have felt reassured. Widgery seemed to care about the things that inform the experience of doctors up and down the country – in areas of social deprivation, certainly, but also throughout the NHS.

Richard Smith believes that medicine, at the beginning of the 21st century, is considered more political than when Widgery was around. Smith blames the lull, a period of stagnation during the second half of the 20th century, which was due to the prominence of a 'silver bullet'; the idea that illness could be cured by a wonder drug (if only it existed) he believes is responsible. Are we to suspect that David Widgery helped to remake the medical political? In some small way, the answer is certainly 'yes'.

Chapter 7

Wider than Widgery

Give me a place to stand, and I will move the world.

Archimedes

The ambition of political doctors must be, in some small way, to move the world. The impression I had when picking up Widgery's work for the first time was, 'Ah, he's cracked it. He discovered the medico-politico equivalent to Archimedes and his lever.' Once you believe something exists, you have the confidence to look again. It became quickly apparent that there were many 'political' doctors. Admittedly this is a rather vague and broad term. Is it possible to define them? There will be many permutations as to what constitutes one. Can they, for example, be recognised by the newspaper they read at lunch time? Or perhaps, less placidly, are they doctors speaking out in the community? Perhaps they simply hold strong ideals about what the world should be like. They come in all shapes and sizes. Some with overlapping features, others with stand alone attributes. And no, they certainly will not all agree.

We have already seen a number of cameos who can be considered political doctors. Our kind conservationists, Iona Heath and Roger Neighbour, with their roles at the Royal College of General Practitioners, are good examples. They are both doctors who seek, in some way, to influence their profession. Iona confesses that becoming a political doctor was not always on the cards. The only reason she was elected to the Royal College was following the positive response she received after having written a letter in anger. There were enough GPs with whom her sentiment struck a chord.

Julian Tudor Hart, the socialist GP from Wales, has established himself as an outspoken political doctor. His research into the inverse care law demonstrated that those areas in Britain with the most wealth received more than their fair allocation of health resources. Born slightly earlier than Widgery, he said, 'I knew exactly what I wanted to do before I left school; to become a general practitioner in a coal mining community ... I might have died in the war, and therefore felt permanently bound not merely to enjoy the peace, but to win and defend it; and not just any peace, but precisely the peace that was won at that time, against Facism and for a new era of the Common Man, as it was said in those days.'[129]

Since then Dr Aneez Esmail has made a mark. In a cunning piece of medical research he proved, along with his colleague Dr Sam Everington, a slice of medical institutionalised racism. By sending off sets of identical junior doctor applications, one with a Western name and another with an Indian name, he found that the latter set were half as likely to be invited for interview.

Where is the best place to stand if you want to exert political change? In a democratic society you might think of parliament. There is a history of doctors becoming MPs. The House of Commons always has one or two scattered on both sides of the house, but not all MD MPs are drawn from established political parties. In 2001 Dr Richard Taylor was elected into parliament on a single issue: the closure of a local hospital. So strong was the local resentment that he removed the Labour candidate with a majority of 17 000 votes.

Having reminded ourselves that there are many political doctors around, we must return to Widgery. Where did his health politics fit into the political spectrum? We will see that the radical revolutionary was not as far from Westminster as his fans might assume. At the same time the beauty of his politics lay in its everyday non-parliamentarian nature.

Political detail

David Widgery in his youth was a radical revolutionary socialist. We have seen that at times he was very anarchic, rejecting traditional radical politics. As a member of IS he was the dissenter. When you speak to people who knew David Widgery, and ask them how they describe their own politics in relation to his, the answer (usually with a few laughs) is that it was impossible not to be to the right.

With his critical voice and his participation in mass movements, Widgery believed that he could change the world. The system could be overthrown and replaced with something else. It would be impossible to say the same of doctors who aspire to get elected into parliament. At the same time, it would be wrong to isolate Widgery from the parliamentary process.

In later life he saw his role as using his voice to pressurise government (even though he dreamed of this different world). In the 1992 film *Utopias* he confesses that, 'We have a different problem from the one Marx and Lenin wrote about in that we have a welfare state. The capitalists decided that they were going to pool all their resources and create the NHS, provide education, etc. We also have a powerful and reformist tradition, which didn't exist in Russia. These two things require of the independent

Left that they are sometimes harshly critical of what the reformists do in the name of socialism.'

This sounds good but there is a problem. Widgery spent the last 13 years of his life under a Conservative government. There was little chance of reforms being passed in the name of socialism. As Turner explained, 'Being a left-wing health worker was a very despairing business. Part of the reason Dave went into medical practice was because he realised that the causes of the Left had been destroyed. He realised that the Left had gone into an unelectable, almost mad position.' There was a feeling that if you really cared for the working class you had to do something to help. Turner continued, 'He could see the way peoples' lives were being destroyed. In terms of unemployment, mortgage rates, in terms of abandonment of the East End, in terms of the lack of investment, in terms of "Who gives a stuff about health unless you've got private health insurance?"'[130]

There was an argument that must have gone, 'oh dear, what's the point of this radical left-wing politics if we are simply allowing the political Right to dominate the power-holding structures?' During the early 1980s Michael Foot was elected leader of the Labour Party, taking them to their worst election defeat since the war. Part of this political disaster is seen to have resulted from a failure to control the far-Left elements in Labour. Turner feels Widgery was dismayed at the consequences of this infighting which allowed Thatcher to walk unchallenged. 'Dave could see that the left-wing coup in the Labour Party had actually been an abandonment of the working classes they were meant to be supporting. In the health context, that's exactly what had happened. If you wanted to look after the people who were turning up on your doorstep increasingly impoverished then you had to think of a more practical way of changing the rules of the game, i.e. gaining power.'

Widgery's ideology may have stayed true but he was not nearly as ambitious as he had been in his youth. Perhaps he became aware of the need to present left-wing views in a format that was palatable in the mainstream. There was no mention of his Socialist Workers Party (SWP) membership in his *BMJ* articles. There is no mention about the need for workers to revolt in his book *Some Lives!*. Could it be that Widgery also discovered that sometimes you have to 'aim a bit around the houses'?

Certainly Widgery became troubled by what he saw in everyday medical practice. Friends feel that he changed as a person. There were two effects; it actually made him gentler and less volatile (something we shall discuss in the next chapter), and it made him question human nature. So overwhelming were the problems encountered that his libertarian approach could not provide a rapid cure. Sue Collinson, neighbour and friend, gives an example of his approach to drug addicts. 'Doing bits and pieces of general practice during the early 1980s Widgery would say, 'Yeah drug addicts. Nice people ... I worked with some in King's Cross.' After a few years of full-time general practice he shifted from an idealised position of 'people doing their own thing, man' towards 'actually they are a nightmare to deal with. They are difficult and I can't solve their problems.'

Trevor Turner suggested that Widgery might even have been something of a New Labour fan. 'He moved away from idealism to a harder understanding about what the health service was about. He didn't dare leave the Left fully, because the Left had been his great cause, but by the end of the 1980s David was very much a Blairite. He was changing, becoming very practical ... What Dave found was that the business of being a doctor, of dealing with people, changed him. He realised that people are not the people left politics take them to be.[130]

Widgery would probably shudder at such comparisons. Even so, the change in his attitudes, which Turner articulates, was not simply one of personal development but a reflection of the change in circumstances that the Left in Britain was facing during the 1980s. Widgery was certainly supportive of the Labour Party as an opposition to the Conservative Party. As Michael Rosen points out, 'that was always the SWP line: "get the Tories out, get Labour in".' The socialist theory is that you go along with the mass movement, then try to radicalise it when in power. Rosen paraphrased Lenin to demonstrate the point, 'Vote Labour with no illusions.'

Rosen reminds us that parliamentary politics was peripheral to the aims of the SWP. For socialists, the workplace was the key. The idea is that workers should determine their own working conditions. If you have powerful enough unions, then you can protect yourself against adverse changes regardless of who holds the parliamentary power. We see this demonstrated by Widgery's actions against hospital closures. If all the hospitals and their workers collectively resisted the changes, Widgery would have argued, they would have been harder to close. Instead they were picked off one by one. In the same way, if teachers, dockers, firemen, etc. all supported each other they would be a power to reckon with regardless of who was in government. Tony Cliff, a prominent member of IS, said in 1970, 'Central to your position is the statement that the emancipation of the working class is the act of the working class – which many only mouth on May Day and other occasions of celebration. This statement is for us the beginning and the end of all our analysis. And if you put the working class at the centre of the arena, then socialism cannot be established except through the expression of the potentialities of the working class.'[131]

It was obvious that during the 1980s things were not good for people on the Left. Turner maintains, 'Dave came to what would be called a middle-of-the-road Labour appreciation. Remember the problem with health politics and being left wing was that we had absolutely no influence on how the Tories decided policy. By definition, if you were left wing, a member of the MPU and making pronouncements about health they would do the complete opposite of what you suggested. By definition, as there was a Thatcherite government in power.' Turner also tells a touching tale of driving home from Thatcher's third successive election win in tears. 'I just wept. Oh no, how much longer is this going to go on? It was just so heartbreaking ... from the point of view of the health service, you could see it being cut and cut and cut.'

Widgery can be interpreted in many ways, just as his *BMJ* columns could be, depending on what the readers' relationship was with him. He was an idealist who wanted to change reality. Undoubtedly he changed as he got older, as did the world. We cannot dispute that his tendency for direct action diminished, his role as a polemic doctor increased. It is interesting that many of Widgery's friends like Fountain and Phillips had, by the 1980s, given up their membership of the SWP. Widgery may have wavered but he never left.

For any political school of thought, there is a need to hold power in central positions (to prevent another camp gaining power) and a need for peripherally located people who are free to speak their minds (to stop the people holding central power forgetting they are there). We can speculate. If Widgery were around and Labour in government, perhaps he would have been a far more effective voice. Trevor Turner thought this was likely, believing that the Labour government might have been happy to have Widgery as an advisor, 'perhaps then we wouldn't have seen Labour make such a mess of health policy, with foundation hospitals for example'.[130]

Medical capital

> The role of the individual advocate underpins all else, but the general practitioner combines this with a wider social and political responsibility to speak out on behalf of the most needy and least heard.
>
> Iona Heath, 1995[132]

Being a general practitioner opened doors for Widgery. It allowed him to appear on television, in newspapers and in books. The result was that he became something of a self-appointed spokesperson for the profession and for the patients he treated. Medicine also provided Widgery with an idealistic trump card. It gave him something to fall back on when other projects were not going too well. To people like Fountain, struggling to become a journalist, Widgery would often turn round and say, 'Huh, what are you doing with your life? I'm a doctor.'

Is there something particular about GPs and political potential? In 1997 Dr Howard Stoate, a GP, was elected as the Labour candidate for Dartford. When interviewed for this book he spoke confidently about the public-political appeal of the general practitioner. 'If you look at any survey, GPs come very near the top of polls in terms of groups in society people listen to, groups people are more likely to go along with. Every time a GP says to somebody that this government has got it wrong, people are far more likely to listen and take it seriously than any other group in society. Governments ignore GPs at their peril.'

For Widgery, the lone libertarian, general practice became the explicit mouthpiece for his ideas. If Widgery had not been a doctor would they have listened? Certainly he would not have had the inspiration for his writing during the late 1980s and 1990s. Widgery is not alone in shaping political argument on medical experience. For example Dr Tonge, a Liberal Democrat MP, stated, 'Good health is not dependent on treatment patients receive from doctors in the NHS but on what politicians do in the field of poverty, housing, and the environment. As an MP I hope I can do something about the reasons people become ill in the first place.'[133] Dr Stoate, who kept up part-time GP surgeries whilst working as an MP, feels medical practice kept him in touch with reality. This, he felt, correlated with political credibility, which had a lot to do with paraphrasing patients' experiences. 'Obviously I change the names. That's why I, even if I say it myself, command a high level of respect in the house. Because people respect a doctor and because I also say, "Well only last week I saw someone in my surgery" ... it goes down very well.'

Calculating what impact Widgery had as an individual is hard. Or perhaps it is simply hard to admit. During the 1980s and early 1990s he probably achieved very little in terms of policy alteration. In fact, it is probably safe to say he failed miserably. Did this mean that he achieved nothing? To answer this question requires us to ask another. How does one make a difference during a lifetime?

Everyday political

The growing good of the world is partly dependent on unhistoric acts; and that things are not so ill with you and me as they might have been, is half owing to the number who lived faithfully a hidden life, and rest in unvisited tombs.

George Eliot, *Middlemarch*

I confessed in the outset that Widgery allowed me to see my own father in a warmer light. One of the letters my family received after his death was from an old schoolfriend of his. Paraphrased, it read something like this: 'I remember he was always full of strong ideals. Perhaps if he had acted on them, the world would be a better place.' During the earlier drafts of this work I would pick my father's mind. Do you wish you were more like Widgery or these other political medics? To which he replied, 'Are they better doctors?'

Widgery's brilliance is that he spoke from a platform of the everyday. Certainly he entertained visions of a grander political work but to many people he was simply that conscientious doctor who cared. Ordinary medical practice requires a political commitment. To look after patients in challenging and profoundly unjust social circumstances is by no means easy. Widgery gave credence to the role of hundreds of everyday GPs and health workers. Without these people, none of the political struggles would matter.

David Widgery inspired people. It is amazing the number of complimentary things people have said during the course of writing this book (although 'Dave was no saint' is also quite popular). A historian must be cynical and say, 'Ah, but they are his friends, or his colleagues ... they are protecting the memory of someone they love and miss. They are protecting themselves, their own understanding of the world.' But every so often you will meet someone who you did not expect to have heard of David Widgery that makes you think, 'His reach was wider than sympathetic East-End GPs and the SWP.' Out of the vagueness of life's encounters you'll meet someone with apparently no reason to remember Widgery. They too will say something equally endearing. This was the case with a newly qualified psychiatrist, which was puzzling because she was too young to have been a doctor when Widgery was around.

'So how do you know him?'
'Oh I heard him speaking on the radio, it was about these Bangladeshi immigrants, his patients were being forced out of their housing by the Docklands development ... Actually he's one of the reasons why I applied to medical school.'

David Widgery may not have succeeded (idealists will always fail) but he made a difference. He reminded many what could be done as a doctor. A sprinkling of faith is required even if the more cynical claim is that it is an illusion.

Chapter 8

Dissecting Widgery

One of the reccuring themes in medicine is hard work. There is no easy option, although you will here whisperings of the latest trend – perhaps it's radiology where, in the future, you can work from home. Supporting this quest for ease is a law that says life must be second place; to do the things you enjoy, to pursue passions that are not directly related to patient care. This is what appears so fantastic about Widgery. He was a journalist, a historian, he organised rock concerts, he was a father and (lest we forget) he was a doctor.

When we stumble across something that appears fantastic we often stare. As inertia passes we may then ask, 'How was that possible?' One of life's greatest challenges is deciding how many objects to juggle and Iona Heath provides a mirror for reflection. Broadly speaking, not wishing to simplify her existence, she chooses to juggle part-time general practice, family life and responsibilities at the Royal College of General Practitioners. Keen to know how she went about this, I asked her about striking a balance. 'If they are all nagging equally then I think I'm doing it right. It's when one starts to predominate and the others nag more, that's when it becomes a problem.' Her son reinforces her diligence, 'She just works bloody hard, Pat.'[132]

It is worth recapping slightly. Iona and Roger paved the way for the tale about a hero. What do we mean by this term? Someone who inspires? Yes. Someone who is perfect? No. This last answer is sometimes hard to accept. Initially my reaction to Widgery was, 'politics, medicine, Hackney, a writer ... brilliant!' Given my predisposing factors, could I be anything but impressed? My medium of discovery is perhaps to blame. Words in print are somehow untouchable. They are there, black against white, neatly folded away from the impingements of everyday life.

The aim of this section is to bring Widgery back down to earth. It would be wrong to provide you with a picture of Widgery rolling through life with infinite ease. All people who have tried to strum the guitar like Hendrix realise that it is harder than it looks. On the other hand, by conveying this difficulty it is hoped that the skill (the art, not the artist) will appear even greater. Even in measured light it is possible to be impressed.

The illusion of everything

Widgery was a journalist, historian, father, GP, campaigner, rock concert organiser, literary critic and friend to many people. Widgery did not do all these things in one smooth motion. To digest his many activities it helps to remember that there were distinct periods of his life. 1968–76: Widgery is doing his medical training, writing for *Oz* and caught up in the humdrum of radical London. 1976–82: Widgery is the newly qualified doctor, located in the East End, fighting the NF with RAR. 1982–92: Widgery has become the family man, pursuing a career in general practice and medical journalism, finding success with *Some Lives!* and the *BMJ*.

So we can see that he did not pack his life into one weekend. At the same time he packed a lot into 45 years. Of interest is how he managed to keep up his medical career at the same time as his wider activities. One answer is 'he didn't'. He hardly went in as a student, he failed his finals and, when he qualified, only did piecemeal general practice. Although later in life he kept up with medicine. He became more committed, taking up full-time general practice, during the last decade of his life. During this time he was still writing books, making documentaries, being a family man and saving local theatres. Were there any strategies Dr Widgery had for doing this?

Widgery was good at managing time. His close friends and colleagues describe a man with an eye on the clock. We shall turn to the deeper reasons behind this later. For the moment let us be content with some general insights. At home Widgery had a special code for those people who wanted to contact him by telephone. This was to filter the political fodder as well as the medical; friends who might be tempted to say, 'Ah Dave, I've got a bit of a sore throat, I was wondering if I could come round and . . .'. If you wanted to contact him and you were permitted to, then you were told the code. Dial the house number, let the phone ring twice and then replace the handset. If you called back immediately, he might answer.

Widgery's life was at times very compartmentalised. It was not just a case of medical practice, political meetings and time for writing. Sometimes people would feel they took second place in the scheme of his busy projects. Anna Livingstone provided the example of her partner, Kambiz, who was extremely excited at the prospect of going out to dinner with his acknowledged hero. 'He left the house effectively saying, "Don't wait up. I'll be back late. Dave and I will no doubt have lots to discuss." He returned crestfallen by half past nine. Widgery had another appointment to attend that evening.'

In the workplace this 'seize the day, get on with things' approach came across. Colleagues described Widgery as very good at 'putting edges on his work,' a skill arguably necessary for time-pressed inner-city GPs. He wrote proficient notes and would often finish surgeries long before others. The downside was that in consultations some patients found him to be abrupt and curt. That Widgery possessed these attributes should not be so surprising.

Widgery described Dr Leibson, his GP mentor to the East End, as 'a medical deviant fiercely independent, blunt to his patients, who none the less admired him'. At the age of 24, Widgery wrote the following about his poetic hero, 'Mayakovosky's communism was, like him, broad shouldered and larger than life, impatient, rude and necessary.'[134]

Widgery could be ruthless with time, which allowed him to fill many compartments but perhaps we are looking at it in the wrong way. General practice in the East End fed into his politics, which fed into his writing. It was, if you like, a perpetual circle – spokes on the same revolutionary wheel. As a doctor he was able to find justification for his wider actions, to check the pulse of an almost global population. Widgery possessed a genuine interest in people and their life stories. Whoever you were, he would want to find out everything about you. This was especially true of the working- class patients he met. He liked nothing more than to listen to a patient who had escaped the Vietnamese Communists or marched alongside the dockers. Speaking for the film *Utopias*, while walking around an East-End estate, he remarks, 'I don't push my politics at all. But I do hope people are open to approaches like that – for example, when I have a patient who's been Jack Jones' right-hand man and we can talk about the dockers, the Pentonville Five and what's gone wrong. Everyone knows something's gone wrong and they want to talk about it. I love that.'

Conflicting interests?

Whether we believe him or not when he says that he does not push his politics, it raises an important question: did having such an explicitly political agenda make his daily medical practice ethically dubious?

Many of Widgery's patients loved that he was so political. They saw him as a champion of their cause. This was certainly the view of Mr Teall, a retired docker, although he admits Widgery seemed more 'extreme' in his views than he and his colleagues had been. If you were being evicted from your flat, you would probably be flattered to see your doctor getting angry on your behalf. Not simply on the end of a telephone, but on national television. At the same time, having a political doctor in the area did not appeal to everyone. The occasional death threat was received by him and his family.

Being politically active enhances the role of the GP. This is certainly the implication of people like Iona Heath, Anna Livingstone and David Widgery. There are perhaps limits to this relationship. It could be argued that Widgery was so successful in his campaigning, certainly in his ability to get his voice heard, that he ceased to be just a political doctor. The role he had carved for himself required more from him than medicine could naturally permit.

It was not uncommon for a colleague to walk into Widgery's room unannounced during the afternoon and find him working, not dictating letters or writing up notes, but on his latest book. Widgery would often be seen to stroll out before everyone else, which could be infuriating for colleagues struggling to get through the day. He might make a political argument about the difficulty of doing smears, but there were some in the practice who felt he should just get on with it.* In other words, whatever your politics the work still has to be done.

Being on call also became a problem for Widgery when, after being stopped by police driving back from a meeting of the SWP in Skegness, he lost his driving licence for refusing to take a breathalyser test. Juliet Ash explained that he had made the journey after being on call the previous night and was given no accommodation. 'After one pint of beer he decided to drive back at one o'clock in the morning. He stopped in a lay-by for some sleep but was woken up by the police. Dave refused to be breathalysed, saying that he could do it himself. He was disqualified from driving for refusing the breathalyser test. It was stupid, but he wasn't drunk.'

The result was that he would sleep in the surgery and carry out visits by bicycle. (This casts a somewhat different light over the depiction of his romantic bus journey to work, as described in the opening chapter of *Some Lives!*)

Highlighting adverse working conditions, while good, is not all good. The documentary *Limehouse Doctor* (produced by the husband of Widgery's sister) made life around the surgery awkward. Film crews are not to be accommodated as inconspicuously as a registrar.† Patients had the excitement of possibly being on television coupled with disappointment if they did not make the cut. But it was Widgery's use of his contacts with patients in the pursuit of wider causes that ruffled most feathers.

---

* Apparent in the practice meeting in the *Limehouse Doctor* documentary.[135]
† GP registrars are doctors training to become fully qualified GPs. Part of their training often involves observing other GPs at work, sitting in on their consultations.

Confidential

The simultaneous appeal and concern regarding *Some Lives!* is that it draws so heavily on the daily experience of David Widgery, the GP. Extracts and descriptions of patient consultations bring the text bubbling to life. For example:

> Ex-docker is a depressive, addicted to tranquillisers. Devoured by his own helplessness which dates from the death of his only daughter in a car accident. A year earlier she had been left by her husband with four children, who subsequently went into care, place unknown. Simultaneous death of his own mother from a painful spleen cancer which required interminable blood transfusions. He has a diarrhoea which no one can explain except as a result of his neurosis.

Or

> A boozer with 'Love' and 'Hate' tattooed on knuckles, stigmata of the Belfast-Glasgow-Teeside lumpen of the industrial crucifixion. Lugged in by a goal-post of a Salvationist. Uncontrolled for nearly 12 years; wine, sherry, Special Brew. 'Anything I can lay my hands on, as early in the day as I can, pissed for breakfast.'

In his defence, Widgery changed the names and many patients were happy when they recognised themselves in the book. Sadly, that's not really the point. It is unlikely that any ethical clearance was obtained or any informed consent given. Some say he simply scribbled notes on the back of prescription pads. Others believed he hid a tape recorder in his drawer.

Think of the local reality. If you happen to live near one of the patients, it does not take much to put two and two together. 'Ah, I know an ex-docker who lives two doors down. He suffers from depression after that awful death of his mother. But did you know he was addicted to tranquillisers? Or that his daughter's husband had left her. How sad his mother dying in that painful horrible way.'

It breaches the Hippocratic oath: 'Whatever, in connection with my professional practice, I see or hear, in the life of men, which ought not be spoken abroad, I will not divulge, as reckoning that all such should be kept secret.' The end may justify the means, but doctors should not be allowed that opportunity in the first place.

Anna Livingstone recalls being particularly outraged by one incident. Around the time of *Some Lives!* Widgery did an interview for *The Sunday Correspondent* supplement to promote his book. Like many such articles it contained some photographs, in this case of Widgery around the surgery. One photograph in particular caused the alarm. It showed the surgery's appointments book lying open. Clearly visible were the names and addresses of some of the patients. Imagine if large numbers of doctors embarked on similar projects? How would you feel if, having visited the doctor two weeks before, you woke up to find your intimate details in a newspaper or best-selling book? You wanted to tell your doctor, not the world. That your name had been changed would be small comfort. People would stop visiting their doctor. Nevertheless following the publication of *Some Lives!*, there was a call for copycat projects from *GP Magazine*. 'Let *GP* reward your observation of Britain today ... We plan a series of articles looking at Britain through GPs' eyes. We want to know what life is like for you and your patients. Is society changing for better or worse?'[136]

A more general and less serious point can be made. Human experience inspires the writer's pen and literary doctors are no exception. Does this cause a problem? Is it necessarily a breach of confidentiality to use material encountered whilst working as a medical practitioner? After all, you do not hear people saying, 'That Doctor Chekhov is a bit out of order. I reckon he got that storyline from one of his own cases.' The defence is that the characters and events are so different in the final version that it would be impossible to tell where they originally came from. Nevertheless this does not provide complete absolution. Doctors who aspire to write often ask themselves, 'Am I a doctor seeing patients or am I a writer looking for material?' It is easy to imagine Widgery answering that question with, 'I'm a doctor first and foremost', but it is tempting to imagine that his true passion was writing. Despite this kind of friction, his colleagues thought he was a charismatic asset to East London primary care. They tolerated his imperfections because they supported the wider things he was involved in.

The impossible task

It is conventional to think of [political] doctors like Ernesto 'Che' Guevara, Norman Bethune and Joshua Horne. But I have more affection for those flaming words of Sylvia Pankhurst (whose mother and baby clinic – a converted pub called 'The Mothers Arms' – was only a stone's throw away from where I practise today) to the judge sentencing her, once again, to jail for sedition: 'I have sat up with the babies all night and tried to make them better. But this is the wrong system and it cannot be made better. And I would give my life to see it overthrown.'[137]

Widgery, to be sure, liked listening to Radio Three, loved his family and was interested in art; but many of his activities outside general practice were hardly an escape from work pressures. Everything in the world could be interpreted through his socialist cognitive schema. Both locally and more globally, he remained adamant that the problems of the world could be resolved if the social structure were changed. It was not a theory he turned to occasionally. This was a way of looking at the world that he lived and breathed. He spent his life trying to change the social model and, at the same time, minimise its harmful effects through his medical practice. The following extract illustrates the dilemma he faced.

It should have been an easy visit, just another case of chickenpox. Some common-sense advice, a bottle of calamine, maybe a squint in the ears, and you can usually be out of the door again in a couple of minutes. This time I was greeted by two kids running barefoot down the length of the council house corridor, naked but for grubby towels, and covered from the soles of their feet to the roofs of their mouths with weeping scabs. Inside, their baby sister lay face down on the carpet like a discarded doll, with a burning fever, rigid neck stiffness, swollen eyelids shut tight over her eyes and with skin almost obliterated with pox craters.

Trying, whilst on the phone, to make light conversation, I asked where Dad was. He was, his wife explained, on remand in Brixton Prison on a charge of attempted murder. Oh, and since he had suffered brain damage in a road accident he was now so deranged that he literally tore his cell apart if not visited every day by his wife. So would I be able to arrange for her to speak calmingly to him over the phone before she accompanied her daughter in the ambulance?

A bad day; we all have them. It only becomes a futile day when I get home and try to unwind in front of the TV set which is celebrating, yet again, that profitless and very expensive venture in the South Atlantic.* I doubt if I have 'saved' more than half a dozen lives in my life, or, to be perfectly honest, prolonged or greatly improved the quality of more than a very few. Yet instead of tackling housing and working conditions, our society has perfected weapons which can blow a cruiser full of teenage conscripts out of the water, which publicly gloats over those boys' deaths and which boasts its ability to blow the entire world into a desert of radioactive dust. What price then the stabilising effect of sodium cromoglycate on mast cells?[137]

During the last ten years of his life medicine and politics were becoming somewhat harmonious. He was enjoying medical practice as a GP with a

* The Falklands War.

cohort of patients, which in turn was inspiring him to write more passionately about the plight of the people he saw. While this might have appeared like a smooth act to outsiders, it was not without rough edges.

One side of Widgery could be extremely charming and professional. He had a strong idea about what a good GP should be like. Like his doctor column in *Socialist Worker*, written under the pseudonym Gerry Dawson, he played the role in the mould of a Balint* doctor with tweed jacket. As Fountain explains, 'He realised that if you are going to relate to the working class from Bow then you behave. You don't bullshit them that you are one of the proletariat. You behave like a good GP, how a good GP should behave.' Dr Zalidis, who worked as a locum at Widgery's practice, certainly remembered him being a charismatic and inspiring presence. (Phillips again recalls the earlier days with Widgery hamming up an East-End accent, trying to communicate to one of his patients they met on the street. 'He put on this phoney Cockney voice, and I thought "Who's he trying to fool?"'.)

Equally, Widgery could be very rude and abusive. This kind of behaviour was most likely to be experienced, not by patients, but by people in Widgery's own peer group. Friends saw his abrasiveness as a defence mechanism. It was a way of protecting himself from the pain he had suffered as a child. Friends tolerated this side of Widgery but, if you were meeting him for the first time, you could be in for a shock.

One day Fountain and Widgery bumped into a woman they had not seen for a while. 'The first thing David said to her was, "Ah, your acne doesn't seem to be anywhere near as bad as it was." And he said it in such a way that the woman looked as though she had been punched. This was a woman who normally answered back.'[20] Such behaviour could be taken as simply 'rude' but it is tempting to look to the reasons behind it.

Searching for clues as to Widgery's drive and more shocking behaviour, we stumble across a recurring theme. Phillips, when asked about the origins of Widgery's idealism, replied, 'He had loving parents, modern house and expensive garden. Maidenhead is cushy at the best of times. I don't know where it came from. Presumably if you have something like polio, there is a sense in which you feel singled out.'[19]

Sheila Rowbotham remembers Widgery being strongly influenced by his childhood neighbours. 'The Thorneycrofts were Communist Party members and upper class intellectuals. Although he admired the Thorneycrofts, he felt they made his mother feel inferior.' Widgery's mother was not apolitical. She was active in the Labour Party, CND, and many progressive Christian causes.

* In 1957 Michael Balint wrote *The Doctor, His Patient and The Illness*,[138] a seminal text about the doctor–patient relationship. Balint groups still meet regularly throughout the country to discuss the issues that arise from their consultations.

Fountain still grapples to understand the impact polio had on Widgery. 'His mother, a devout Christian, loved Widgery, but he was atheist in a really violent way. I've thought about it after the event. I thought it was due to David's sense of resentment – "Mother, you had all these ideas and I was in all this pain." I think this produced the part of Widgery that was staggeringly rude. It produced the belief that doctors cure people. It also produced the snappy tone of voice with which he would say, "What are you bothering about? Don't worry about the petty things. Get on with the important things."'[20] Rowbotham feels that while Widgery reacted against his mother's goodness overtly, he was inwardly very close to her.

Widgery's isolation from a society he simultaneously loved and loathed was heightened by education. The 1950s grammar school provided nourishment for the seeds that were beginning to germinate thanks to works by Russell and Shaw. Looking back, Widgery reflected on this period that was to reach a climax when he was expelled for publishing a sexually explicit magazine.

> The school I attended was one of that dying breed, the grammar school-with-pretensions. It was the last Grammar School Show, an educational version of *Hancock's Half-hour* where a rather seedy group of teachers, who clearly felt themselves destined for higher things, attempted to bully some culture into a group of roughs who were much more interested in motor bikes and Bert Weedon's 'Guitar Tutor' and 'getting off with birds' – as we described our largely imaginary sexual efforts.
>
> The staff attempted to provide airs for their graceless pupils and had inherited an honours board in oak and gilt (although only a handful only ever made it to university), a school song in cod-Latin (which had a couplet about the school's lofty position over the railway sidings) and a panelled headmaster's study (where the head would beat you with a strap and show you his holiday slides of the Panthenon on successive days).
>
> The masters had bicycles and wore mysterious gowns on speech day, but for all the imitation-public schoolery it was still run on exams, intimidation and competition, where we remained dumb and as insolent as possible.[139]

Medical school can only have heightened this sense of not quite belonging. At the same time he was a rebel floating in the mainstream. Widgery, like most of us, was not without contradictions. For an anarchist he could be quite authoritarian. As Phillips recalled, 'There was this side to David. He did like people who were authorities in their field, like expert historians. For someone who got expelled from school, there was a part of David that was a kind of headmaster. He would see you as falling short by some kind of standard, as not measuring up to authority.'[19] This paradox is captured in his disgust for Classic FM (commercial easy listening) in favour of Radio Three (government funded for the connoisseur), 'I'm for republican excellence against market-led levelling down, and if that makes me Reithian,* too bad.' Fountain reckoned that while Widgery was 'motivated by a deep and corrosive and wonderful loathing for the British class system or for British society as it was', he was nevertheless 'indeed deeply English.'[20]

While Widgery's ideals were strong, they were not always overriding. During the 1980s he and his friend Trevor Turner developed a professional partnership. Widgery would call Turner and say, 'I've got another one!' Together they would travel to certify the dead body, receiving a fee known as 'ash cash'. To the restaurant they would go, to wine and dine at the expense of the dead.

Fountain reflects that Widgery was permitted a certain freedom. 'David came from a group of people who listened to *Hancock's Half-hour*. Attending a grammar school, there was that sense of displacement. There's a bunch of public school snobs, you're not one of them. That was one of the reasons why he was attracted to people like Richard Neville, the founder of *Oz* magazine. An Australian, Neville could go for rides in the British class system because he was not part of it.'[20]

Dabbling in excess

At various points in his life Widgery indulged in too much alcohol and drugs. There are many reasons for this. Partly he was a child of the 1960s and 'well, didn't everyone?' Marijuana and LSD were common in the social circles he frequented during the early 1970s. As he wrote in *Oz*, 'LSD's profoundly disinhibitory effect on the sensory nervous system was expressed in the synaesthetic subjectivity of much of the best design and a kind of political pantheism which was both idiotic and divine. And if a staple diet of cannabis sometimes produced fatuous thought, it did not produce the anergia of heroin.'

Drugs can react differently in different people. Widgery, often to the amusement of friends, gained himself a reputation for being a lightweight. There would come a point, usually after a couple of glasses of wine, where Widgery would be drunker than most. Phillips and Fountain felt he had great powers of autosuggestion. As students, they rolled him a joint of marijuana containing only tobacco. Widgery still got stoned. Peer

---

* John Reith was the first Director General of the BBC.

pressure? There were more bizarre examples during his student days.

Widgery had been to a Rolling Stones concert and drunk too much. Fountain and his girlfriend at the time were responsible for his safe return. 'We had to get him in a taxi at Piccadilly, which took about an hour and a half. My girlfriend was petite, and I'm no Charles Atlas. When we did get him into a cab, back to Chapel Market, we dragged him upstairs. He was completely out of it. We started walking down the stairs. As we did so, we heard Widgery get up and go over and put on his record player.'[20]

In the context of artistic expression, tapping into the imagination with drugs is nothing new. Widgery's heroes like Ginsberg and Kerouac were heavily into LSD. We would do well to remember that many authors found space on shelves marked 'Classics' thanks to a drug named opium. At various times in his life Widgery injected substances. While it is impossible to understand exactly why he did this, there is a strong feeling that this was part of his 'shocking' tactics. Friends have postulated it was a way of showing he was stronger than his polio, as well as numbing the pain.

This element of Widgery's life is especially shocking when we think of the clean-cut medical practitioner.

Michael Rosen recalls Widgery explaining his creative view of the world. '"You can only tolerate the extremes you are putting yourself through, by courting with a certain extremism or insanity." Dave was fascinated and intrigued by that kind of "push yourself to the edge and go". That was how you coped with the system. His great hero was Peter Sedgwick, who went early as well. How this ties in with medicine is fascinating. The tradition of the lefty doctor is so far from Shelley and Rimband or Charlie Parker blowing his brains out. Widgery was interested in all this. He would take the piss out of me for being "straight". The irony was that I was the writer and he was meant to be the doctor.'

A deeper sense of time

The more aware you are of time, the more you value it. People who have had near-death experiences often go on to achieve remarkable things. Widgery certainly had a close experience with death as a child, when he was diagnosed with polio and later with TB. These were experiences that scarred him more than many people appreciated. They had a profound impact on Widgery as a person, causing him great pain and suffering.

Polio was not an illness readily cured. The operations he received as a child allowed him to walk, but not to run. Juliet Ash describes how he was 'incredibly shy about his physical disability and at times both hurt and amused when kids would mimic his lop-sided walk'. In many ways

Widgery compensated with his charisma, flamboyant confidence and success in many spheres of life. Did Widgery have something to prove during his life? If he did, and most humans do, it was a task heightened by his illness. This had a great deal to do with time.

Widgery's polio left him in intermittent pain. It also left him worried that he would not be able to continue and would end up in a wheelchair. Not long before his death he alluded to this.

> No, I still haven't come to terms with it. I don't think I will for a while. I get long periods when I forget about it, but as I get older I do get more fatigued ... Last night I was humping three bags of medical equipment round an estate in Bow, getting lost and having to climb lots of stairs. I got halfway up the second lot, I was terribly tired and my back was hurting – I've got a bit of a back problem because of the asymmetry – and I suddenly thought, 'I'm in my mid-forties and I don't like the look of this. I won't be able to do this in ten years' time.' You suddenly realise that the sort of mental energy that a lot of people who've had polio, or other kinds of illness, manage to acquire is going to be drained by the physical weight you're having to carry, that you probably won't live as long as everybody else, that you'll get more exhausted more quickly, that you'll probably get home-bound, or chair-bound, or bed-bound sooner.[140]

In this light, some of the conversations we see during *Limehouse Doctor* take on greater significance. Partners at the practice are shown discussing the need to perform more cervical smears. Widgery argues that after talking to a patient, there is simply not enough time. 'I'm obsessive about not getting behind time. You have a long conversation, then do the smear, put it on the computer, write on the slide. I can't do it under 12 minutes. I feel like you're fighting a battle with time. You've got thousands of trampling feet out there waiting to see you. I'm scared, neurotically scared of getting behind time. I'm fighting with time to stay on time.'[135]

The meaning is deeper than that which most GPs would understand. As Phillips reflected on Widgery when he was in his twenties, 'One of the things I found most bizarre was that he could never relax in the bath. It wasn't as though he was a twitchy sort of person. It was because he couldn't waste the time. He was attracted to people like Billie Holliday and Dylan Thomas. He was interested in these meteoric wild people who lived to the limit. By willpower, by the sheer force of their creativeness. These kinds of people can be fascinating and a complete pain. They thrive to an extent off the people around them. They create space; they need breathing space.'[19]*

---

* As Kerouac wrote, 'mad to live, mad to die, burn, burn, burn like fantastic candles across the night sky'.

Nigel Fountain remembered one of the last times he heard Widgery's voice. 'We were at this party. David was saying to this kid, "You've got to stick up for yourself. Don't let other people drag you down. Get in there first." This was one of the reasons why David was so phenomenally rude.'[20] Fountain thinks Widgery's forthrightness was 'probably a defence mechanism. It was a "You mustn't get near me. Don't insult me. Fuck off. Leave me alone." So you hit them so bloody hard they were gaping.'[20]

Widgery pursued passions with vigour. Something demonstrated by his taste in music. Whilst others were content to keep their Rolling Stones records, Widgery became part of the punk scene. Later in life he listened to classical music. Turner explains, 'Dave had to listen to the whole god damn thing, not just the nice slow movements.' A philosophy personified by the fact that he listened to the whole Verde Corpus four years before he died. (This boundless enthusiasm could, at times, be blind; Widgery would often pursue debates with Juliet Ash about art, believing that he held the best understanding when in fact she was the expert.)

When Widgery got involved in a project, he injected energy. The late Paul Foot (a prominent figure in the SWP) reiterated something similar to Michael Rosen in his creative view of Widgery, 'David was a restless man. He was always driving his body further than it could go in feverish pursuit of something unattainable.' Was Widgery a modern-day romantic?

Time is everything, as Widgery infers in the film *Utopias*. 'I think working with ill people and working with people in crisis puts a microscope on life. You do see things more intensely. And you see choices and possibilities and difficult decisions magnified. That heightens your awareness of what life's about. It heightens your awareness of how quickly we are getting older, how little time we have on this planet, how much there is to be done, and how easy it is to waste time.'

From such a perspective the imperfections of Widgery fade away. In the scheme of things, perhaps having patients' names and addresses appearing in a newspaper was not that important.

Pushing out bridges

Towards the 1990s Widgery had become more indulgent. He appeared to be drinking more than was good for him. As the socialist historian David Renton recounts, 'by the 1980s Widgery's illness was clearly much worse. He admitted to Ruth Gregory that he was in a lot of pain, a lot of the time. He drank more, and smoked, and was often rude (or worse) when drunk. According to his friend Syd Shelton, "he knew no moderation in anything".'[141]

Juliet Ash felt Widgery put up with a great deal of pain in later life. He was deeply tired. He possessed a stoicism that said, 'you get on with things', to the extent that few people knew how much he suffered. For us, it is perhaps impossible to imagine.

Fountain believes that Widgery was afraid. Nigel Fountain believed that 'part of David was actually terrified. Terrified that he wasn't as good as people thought he was. He was as good but he was terrified of it. What he did in the later stages of his life was swing from productive work to anni- hilation. By the beginning of the 1990s I think David was under strain because he was thinking, "I've now got to start coming out with some thoughts here, some work, I've really got to come out and do this." He was very rigorous; he worked very hard and had absolute manic periods of activity. But that would then be followed by "I'll disappear or get pissed". That was the kind of tightrope he was walking.'

In late 1992 Widgery was preparing to take his sabbatical at the Wellcome Institute. He was very excited at this prospect as it would allow him to highlight the chaos that had existed before the foundation of the NHS. It was none other than Roy Porter who had asked Widgery to write his history of East-End medicine.

On the night of 26 October 1992 David Widgery died. He had taken a number of substances, including alcohol, barbiturates and injected pethi- dine. The primary cause of death was found to be asphyxiation. Newspapers later reported the story of a druggie doctor who had died from an overdose. Friends and family felt this was a gross misrepresenta- tion. The shock of his untimely death was heightened by the disbelief that this could have happened at all.

Professional colleagues had no inkling that this might be on the cards. There was no question about Widgery's competency to perform as a doctor; colleague contact and practice audits never suggested anything sub-standard. Anna Livingstone reflected fondly that, 'we had no idea that he might do this ... but then he did fall off the roof once when trying to fix it'.

Death is not a pleasant thing. People were greatly angered that Widgery should have allowed himself, coining a phrase used by many, 'to be so bloody stupid'. Friends find it sadly ironic that Widgery lived like his romantic heroes more than was necessary. His writings are littered with examples, almost predictions of his own exit. For example, he wrote for *Oz* in 1969, 'Now Cassady's dead too. His body was found beside a railroad track outside the town of San Miguel de Allende in Mexico. It was said that he had been despondent and felt that he was growing old and had been on a long downer and had made the mistake of drinking alcohol on top of barbiturates. His body was cremated.'

There are many theories about what exactly happened. For us, who did not know or love Widgery, they can be no more than idle speculation. If we are to refer to anything it must be the coroner's report and its open verdict. A *BMJ* review of the television programme *Limehouse Doctor* (screened after his death) provides some pertinent words.

Not all viewers will share the uncritical idealism with which David Widgery appeared to view the plight of his down-trodden, homeless patients, but few will fail to be impressed by the tenderness with which he ministered to them or the passion with which he championed their cause. Those who work in the high stress environment of inner city primary care will, in retrospect, recognise signs of Widgery's escalating exhaustion towards the end of the programme. The coroner reached an open verdict, but, one way or another, Widgery's commitment to the people of Limehouse was the death of him. Did he, in his short life, achieve even a measurable fraction of the impossible task he had set himself? Perhaps not, but in the words of one of the winos who watched his coffin disappear down the litter strewn street, "Holy God, he was one hell of a doctor".[142]

1992 for David Widgery, the historian, GP, polemicist, father and campaigner, should have been the beginning. Not the end.

Chapter 9

Concluding a radical life

The Talmud tells how a rabbi was once passing through a field and saw a very old man planting an acorn. 'Why are you planting that?' he asked. 'You surely do not expect to live long enough to see the acorn grow up into an oak-tree?' 'Ah,' replied the old man, 'my ancestors planted trees not for themselves, but for us, in order that we might enjoy the shade of their fruit. I am doing likewise for those who come after me.'

Summary

Chapter 2 outlined how I came to write about David Widgery. I explained my environmental (being a slightly disgruntled medical student) and genetic (having a dad as a GP) predisposition. I stated that his life had inspired me by demonstrating that doctors can concern themselves with wider issues, as well as practising medicine as it is traditionally understood.

In Chapter 3 you saw how David Widgery embraced life on many fronts, creating identities in different worlds. He was a political writer for *Oz*, the 'charismatic leader figure' of the IS, the failed saviour of East-End hospitals, the invisible medical student, the enemy of the NF, a catalyst for conscientious punk music, a loving father, the committed East-End GP and an outspoken *BMJ* columnist. These elements fused during the 45 years he was alive.

Chapter 4 was a reminder about the social causes of ill health. It pointed out that the social causes are often sidelined. This can be a cause of disillusion, one that socialist doctors perhaps acknowledge more so than others. We looked at Widgery's idealism in relation to his medical career choice; we saw that he was not the only doctor to share similar sentiments.

Medicine seemed at times like a distant commitment for Widgery, but this changed as he grew older. He found he was able to strike a balance between his writing, his politics and his medicine. Skills learnt as a political-journalist-activist, as we saw in Chapter 5, were applied to the medical workplace. Engaging with the channels before him, he attended meetings, occupied hospitals, wrote letters to defend housing claims and argued for individual hospital beds. In the late 1970s he occupied Bethnal Green Hospital in an unsuccessful attempt to prevent its closure.

I have argued that outside interests (idleness) might be important in making happier (better) doctors. Chapter 6 explored the particularly close relationship writing (as a form of idleness) has with the medical profession – both as a tool for understanding and a means of expression.

David Widgery from a young age, isolated in hospital wards with polio, developed a taste for literature. Having surveyed his career as a journalist in the wider world, we looked at how his writing was applied to the world of medicine. Widgery's passion and belief in the need for an NHS cannot be doubted. *The National Health* pointed out, with historical perspective, many of the problems facing the health service in 1988, but was not too clear how to improve things. It should be noted that Widgery was not always accurate or honest.

Some Lives! was the pinnacle of his writing. It was a vivid portrayal of the reality he experienced as a doctor that won him widespread acclaim. More so because of the problems the Docklands development, which Widgery was opposed to, was facing at the time. His column in the *BMJ* reflected the success he was gaining as a medical journalist. It allowed him to reflect and report on the impact of government policy on both doctors' and patients' lives. This struck a chord with many doctors.

Chapter 7 showed that political doctors act in many ways. Reminding ourselves of this diversity, we then proceeded to look at how Widgery changed his approach with age. Moving away from a radical socialist approach to a politics that engaged more with central government. While some people see Widgery as a political entity separate from medicine, I have argued that his power stemmed from the role of Dr Widgery. His appeal stemmed greatly from the appearance of the everyday GP, working in adverse conditions many 'everyday political' doctors recognised.

Chapter 8 shows us that Widgery was not a model of perfection. While many patients liked him, there were also those who found him impatient and rude. Did his wider projects compromise his position to practise everyday medicine? Breeching medical confidentiality would suggest that at times they did. Widgery did struggle about what to do with his life. Was it best to be a doctor? Was it better to be politically engaged outside medicine? For someone who wanted to see so much change, the world was a frustrating place. Friends described how Widgery's polio shaped his outlook on the world. Perhaps there was a feeling of being second best that drove him on to try as hard as he did. We have touched lightly on the subject of his drug experimentation. Although drugs may not have played a part in his later life, they played a part in his tragic death.

It is tempting to wonder what would have happened to David Widgery, had he lived longer. There are some who believe that he would have gone from strength to strength, writing more effectively for a wider and wider audience. As friends lamented, *Some Lives!* should have been the turning point in his career not the end. In this sense his medical practice might have subsided, as it was about to for his year's sabbatical shortly before his death, the juggling act between the two arenas becoming increasingly difficult to balance. Trevor Turner suggests that New Labour, in a tactical move to keep hold of the Left's grass roots, might have recruited Widgery as an advisor on health. On the other hand, many of Widgery's close friends would react angrily to such an affiliation. Sheila Rowbotham stresses how disappointed Widgery would have been with the Blair Project, which 'has been so hostile to issues of class inequality'. She draws our attention to Labour's intervention in the public sector, which are 'terribly managerial and top-down; they are designed to exert control and do not foster real choice at all'.

We can be certain Widgery would not have clapped the arrival of Public Finance Initiatives and another war in Iraq.

I personally imagine that a better-balanced Widgery would have done part-time general practice, using the other time to develop his writing further. It is difficult to imagine him abandoning medicine completely, as this was the public identity (Widgery, the doctor) which he had successfully established for himself. He would probably be singing the praises of the Hackney Empire, campaigning for more from the Mayor of London and dismissing any politician who dared to pass judgement on the NHS.

A life cannot be easily proved or refuted. What lessons are taken away from David Widgery will vary. For this reason, I shall close as I started, by speaking about those things I believe to be especially important.

Thought provocation

David Widgery's life provokes many questions. Ultimately I believe they boil down to the following.

- What is the role of the doctor in society?
- How can doctors fight for their ideals in medico-political arenas?
- How can doctors be happier?

These are the questions that initially drew me towards David Widgery. They have shadowed the words I subsequently wrote. What then are the answers?

When I picked up his book *Some Lives!* four years ago in the studious atmosphere of the Cambridge University library, I genuinely thought that answers did exist. I thought that if I could get a grip on what David Widgery was like, how he went about tackling his frustrations, I would have the solution in my hands. Then I might be able to spread this message to hard-working GPs like my dad. Happiness, joy and laughter would prevail and the medical profession would be a better place.

The more I looked the more complicated it became. Firstly, it turned out that David Widgery did not even want to be a GP, he wanted to be a writer. Then it turned out that not everybody liked him as a person, that he could be slightly annoying. Worst of all, I began to realise that perhaps David Widgery was not the doctor for me to be. Could it be that I was not as radical as my Jimi Hendrix poster led me to believe? I became confused.

Having set such a mammoth task for David Widgery, failure was inevitable. But his failings were not absolute. Overcoming my mistaken idolisation I began to see Widgery in a more measured light. Writing has allowed me to digest these questions, even if they remain impossible to answer.

His/her story

Medicine and the business of being a doctor are far from static. Much that those in the present take for granted was once contested. Not all surgeons in the 19th century said, 'Ah, bacteria, why didn't you say so? I'll scrub my hands then'. On the contrary, some were very sceptical. 'Where are these little beasts.' rasped John Hughes Bennett, professor in Edinburgh. 'Show them to us and we shall believe in them. Has anyone seen them yet?'[56]

Widgery had a wonderful sense of history. He believed that the past shaped the present, that the present shaped the future. This conviction empowered him. For example, by the early 1990s Widgery saw great similarities between the changes he was witnessing in the NHS and the 'chaos out of which the health service was created' a century before. 'We have a situation where hospitals are under siege and GPs are in competition with each other. It's a bit like looking into some ghastly mirror and recognising your own face.' This perspective made him more determined about the need to oppose the introduction of the internal market.

David Widgery demonstrates that doctors can think about the past and that this appreciation can feed into the role they pursue in the present. Mark Bloch, who was executed during World War II for helping the French Resistance, wrote a charming book called *The Historian's Craft*. He articulates something of the passion that brings people to study history, a subject that is considered by many to be dusty and irrelevant. There is an extract worth sharing.

> Misunderstanding of the present is the inevitable consequence of igno-
> rance of the past. But a man may wear himself out just as fruitlessly in
> seeking to understand the past, if he is totally ignorant of the present ...
> I had gone with Henri Pirenne to Stockholm; we had scarcely arrived,
> when he said to me: 'What shall we go to see first? It seems that there is
> a new city hall here. Let's start there.' Then, as if to ward off my
> surprise, he added: 'If I were an antiquarian, I would have eyes only for
> the old stuff, but I am a historian. Therefore I love life.'[143]

Doctors do not have enough time to become fully fledged historians (although I am sure some might enjoy it). Instead doctors should perhaps be encouraged to occasionally glance back at the past, in the same way non-astronomers can still appreciate the stars. At every moment there has existed debate about what medicine is, about what the doctor should be doing, about the kind of system that provides healthcare. This has an empowering implication because it tells us that the future has not been written. Debates that happen now matter.

Iona and Roger encourage us to search far and wide for heroes and hero-ines. This is necessary because medical heroes, we might argue, cause unhappiness. This paradox reflects that to become a doctor requires people to think alike. Heroes, usually in the form of oil on canvas, stare boldly out into the ether of time. They are there to show us how it is done. While we may learn to appreciate the brilliance of keeping an eye on water pumps in Soho and occasionally dream about sailing a ship called *The Beagle*, these role models are a variation on a theme. We are taught to aspire towards the great men of science, the forefathers of our concrete present. We must realise that science is just a factor in the medical equation.

Perhaps we need to create a more balanced view between the sciences and the arts. Whether or not this is something that can be encouraged by institutions alone is difficult to say. Some medical schools run creative writing courses or encourage the reading of literature. From my experi-ence, reading and writing provide a refreshing complement to medical education. Perhaps we might encourage more applicants into medicine who are keen to help people but remain deterred by the idea that chem-istry is the shape of things to come.

Trevor Turner seems to believe something similar, 'We are desperately in need of more articulate doctors. We need more Daves, no doubt about it. Part of the problem with medicine is that because it's become so popular it is forced into taking people with A-plus pluses straight across the line, instead of what we might call 'characters'. Part of the reason for the professor being so demoralised today is that we have these superstar people, with As in physics, chemistry and maths, going into a profession that does not require that kind of ability.'

Social inequalities

Social inequalities and health inequalities remain. They continue to impact on the role of the health professional. Should the doctor therefore be tackling the social causes of ill health? If the answer is 'yes', then maybe there is a need for a more explicit role, as Tudor Hart claims: 'If social factors influence the behaviour of disease on a community-wide scale, GPs and other primary care workers must concern themselves with them as a normal and central part of their work, not as a fringe option to be added by some doctors and ignored by others.'[144]

The difficultly is that there is no silver bullet. Problems like racism, poverty and poor housing are too big for the doctor to alone to tackle. Equally they are too big for doctors to ignore. Widgery's actions stand out but he believed them to be part of a wider social scheme. He regarded them as collective problems, in which his voice was one among many. This had a lot to do with his socialist outlook on the world.

Critics may say, 'Well, whether or not he was a doctor he would have been fighting for redistribution of wealth. Medicine was him hijacking another socialist cause.' There is some truth to this statement. Indeed Le Fanu, a writer of popular medical books, believes health inequalities are a problem of relative poverty not absolute poverty. 'Behind the guise of being scientific and objective, it [The Black Report] is a political document that seeks to bolster the arguments for radical reform by portraying the class divisions in society within the terminology of health.'

This is a difficult statement to defend against – one that could lead to a regression of despair. Does true objectivity exist? Can a scientific paper be free from politics? Even if it is created in the world of neutrality, does this not evaporate as soon as it's read? Socialist or not, I believe there are many doctors who would argue that redistribution of wealth would help their patients' health. Does the fact that Tudor Hart is a socialist discredit the inverse care law? The role of ideology in medical practice is an interesting one.

We might argue that it is not the place of a doctor to grind a political axe. Some would point out that all axes, when held up to the light, glint with a political edge. In my father's consultation room he had placed a big *Evening Standard* placard in one corner, altered to read, 'REFUGEES ARE WELCOME HERE'. Was this wrong? The tabloids were implying that most asylum seekers were bogus, which in his opinion was helping to further ostracise many vulnerable people in East London. Certainly it must be on a footing with other instances of politics in the workplace. Doctors often conduct research into relatively rare conditions, conditions that would benefit from greater recognition and financial backing. It is not unheard of for them to make a political case to their patients: 'It would be better if the government gave us more money, why don't you get active?' Encouraging a more tolerant view of refugees, when a doctor believes this would benefit patients, falls into the same category. To what extent does the neutrality of the doctor hold strong?

So much goes unsaid in medicine. One of the best bits of advice I received for my application to medical school was, 'Every time you look in the mirror say to yourself, "Why do I want to practise medicine?"' Successful candidates, medical students and therefore doctors, should not stop asking this question. I believe it would make for a healthy exercise. If we understand why we are here, perhaps we will better understand where we are trying to go.

Confronting an ill society is not an easy task. It requires a different kind of commitment, one that has to be balanced with medical responsibilities, family and relaxation. David Widgery was busy even by doctors' standards. Perhaps there are other role models of moderation from which to learn. At the same time we should remember to judge Widgery with a pinch of salt. He did not ask us to peer into his life. Nor did he claim to have all the answers. Friends loved him because he could 'light up the night sky' and had the 'power to illuminate, shock and delight'.

Widgery's life demonstrates how difficult the battle for healthcare can be. He had to fight long and hard for resources, usually with minimal success. It often felt as though he were banging his head against a brick wall. The louder he shouted, the more he hoped people would listen. This might appear crude but it is indicative of a Balkanised health system. There are many separate groups, all with potentially competing interests. Consultants have different interests from GPs, who have different interests from nurses, who all have different interests depending on which part of the country they work in. Widgery believed his causes deserved attention but he also knew that you had to make an argument for them. He drew strength from a belief that his patients and colleagues were especially hard done by. They were already poor and working in depressing circumstances. The last thing they needed were changes making life more difficult. So while everybody in the health service warrants sympathy and more money, it might be argued that Widgery's causes deserved them more than most. This is not to say that he did not possess a wider view, merely that he thought taking a narrow and extreme view was a necessary tactic.

The problems faced in deciding the allocation of resources within the NHS are the same as those facing any democracy. You want it to be representative but this is impossible unless people speak up. Sometimes it takes a character like Widgery to give them a voice.

Health advocates

David Widgery believed in the NHS. Knowing that someone thinks similar thoughts can be immensely important, especially if you feel they are becoming increasingly marginalised in the public arena. The NHS continues to be perceived and perpetuated by many as a failure. For this reason Widgery's voice remains fresh and invigorating. 'In the 1980s, politically dominated by the philosophy of possessive individualism, the NHS still allows a different set of values to flourish.'

In 1988 Julian Tudor Hart wrote, 'We have to make a start from where we are with the people we have. The NHS contains elements of a future more equitable, stable, happier society on which we can build. In the minds of the people it remains a successful demonstration of the superiority of service for need over commodity production for profit.'[144]

The NHS needs advocates like Tudor Hart and Widgery. Otherwise we risk forgetting why the NHS exists at all. We could paraphrase the Feynman quote I used at the outset, 'In religion, the moral lessons are taught, but they are not taught once – you inspire again and again, and I think it is necessary to inspire again and again, and to remember the value of the NHS [substituted for science] for children, for grown-ups and everybody else.'[11]

Ideas need to be sold. This was something Widgery was extremely good at, demonstrated by RAR. He believed that culture could be used for good and for bad. Everywhere we look there are examples. As these words are written, the drive to recruit more teachers in the UK is being helped by adverts portraying the profession as awe inspiring. The catch phrase is 'Those Who Can Teach'. So good are these adverts you almost want to leave the cinema, skipping the film, and say, 'Yes. I can. I'd love to teach. Let me help them to make a better world.' The NHS has great potential to match such efforts. People do not need converting. They need reminding – something that Widgery was very good at.

The principle of universal healthcare has run into some serious difficulties since it was conceived: the ageing population, the spiralling cost of treatment, increasing public expectations and drug resistance have all played a part. Widgery was guilty of at times taking a simplistic view.

People who defend the NHS should remember that dreams need to be realistic if they are to be accepted as solutions. Similarly those who get caught up in the nitty-gritty of health politics should not lose sight of the bigger picture.

I too believe that health needs to be thought of as a collective problem. Since Widgery's death in 1992, life has become increasingly medicalised. Existence, and all that it entails, is seen to have a medical cause and thereby a potential medical cure. This makes the NHS's predicament logically untenable, the role of the GP who must filter the ocean . . . impossible.

We do need to decide what the NHS can and cannot do. This a call, not for radical measures, but to pause and take a deep breath. What does the NHS do well? What can it do better? In what ways can people help it to stay alive and function to the best of its ability? Do we automatically think that the grass is greener elsewhere in the world? If we had to choose our flaws, and we must choose some, what would they be?

In 2002 the NHS Confederation published a document entitled, *'The problem of unhappy doctors – what are the causes and what can we do?'*. 'Doctors are not trained in a way that prepares them for the messy and complex world of organisations. In particular they are often not given the opportunity to learn the skills and behaviour necessary to engage with organisations which could do much to help them with the sources of dissatisfaction.'[145] This sounds very Widgery. Most telling was a call for doctors to step out into the wider world. 'The media and politicians play a key role in shaping consumers' expectations of their doctors, and therefore this is the hardest area to influence. . . . There is a need to be more open about the limits of medicine, to resist the tendency to medicalise aspects of ordinary life and to continue to reinforce the message that citizens need to take responsibility for their own health. A much more proactive attempt to engage the media, politicians and public is required if this is to succeed.'[146] Perhaps they are suggesting, ten years after Widgery's death, that more doctors should confront a society that shapes ill health.

The doctor's role

A great tragedy has occurred if the role of the doctor is to be overworked, tired and full of regret. The impression I got from my father, speaking to other GPs, junior doctors, consultants and just generally keeping my ears open, is that lots of these emotions are compounded by a sense of powerlessness. Doctors often feel overwhelmed by the social problems they have to confront. They also feel unable to influence government policy to say, 'I don't agree, listen to me'. Dr James Willis argues in *Friends in Low Places* that, 'we should not underestimate the importance of giving people the idea that they could make a difference'.[147]

Where does the responsibility of the doctor lie? Is it with individual patients or is it engaging in the wider system? Most people would quickly argue for the former, yet Widgery reminds us that the two realms are not mutually exclusive. If the causes of patients' problems lie outside the consulting room, then perhaps doctors need to be doing more of the latter, becoming advocates for their patients in the wider sense, as *The Mystery of General Practice*[132] encourages. Equally, doctors need to look out for themselves.

David Widgery was remarkable, but it is hoped that he appears accessibly ordinary. He wrote letters, attended meetings and scribbled words, organising them systematically on sheets of paper. Widgery was undoubtedly happier because of these actions; he believed that what he did outside the consultation room could affect what happened within it. He was not always successful but he tried. And while there are examples of other similarly engaging doctors, Widgery possessed more passion than most. Powerless doctors could (if they so choose) use their voice to challenge an undesirable policy.

Turner was particularly struck by Widgery, 'I do not believe that doctors can be in the frontline seeing patients all the time, no doubt about it. That's why I'm amazed at what GPs do. I think they do too much frontline work. You have to see your patients and do your clinical activities but you've also got to have other things to distract you from the hurly-burly otherwise you get bored, burnt out and fed up. Some people do this by research, others by writing. Only way to be a good doctor is not just to see patients, you have to think how can you help things in the broader context.'

Widgery's life does carry a subversive message. Doctors should be happy. Perhaps this was because Widgery did not live a life of straight lines. He chased dreams blindly and enthusiastically. Dreams that (thankfully for the purposes of this book) potentiated the experience he had with his patients and community. I personally find that wonderfully inspiring. Nor am I alone. David Renton wrote, 'Such adjectives as "Epicurean" or Samuel's "Dionysian" capture the sense of a man who consistently supported play over work, joy over guilt, and the pleasure of life as it could be, over the misery of life as it was.'

General practice

We must be generalists acknowledging all forms of distress as legitimate, and we need to be able to provide continuity of care over time ...

A grasp of philosophy and politics can show us how to be effective partisans on behalf of our patients.

Iona Heath[132]

General practice in the United Kingdom changed during the second half of the 20th century. The drive to improve standards, along with the mounting pile of paperwork required to do this mean that people no longer enjoy the job as they once did. Early retirement appears to be the hassle-free option. At the other end of the age spectrum, a new generation of GPs prefers the freedom of locum work. As Neighbour points out, it is a self-perpetuating problem. With short-term contracts, continuity of care disappears and it becomes impossible to develop the kind of relationship that so many GPs have previously valued. The job becomes a bore.

Looking at Widgery cannot solve a recruitment problem. Nevertheless it is hoped that policy makers will remember why so many people have found general practice appealing; continuity of care, belonging to the local community, spending time with patients (things that Widgery articulated well).

David Widgery's writing fuels the fire of those who feel standards are clouding things that cannot be quantified. As Dr Paul Julian, an East-End GP not far from retirement reflected after reading an earlier draft of this work, 'what has happened to the magic we experience when we peer into people's lives?' People represent much more than data points. Doctors spend more and more time being told to look narrowly by directives, searching for things that eclipse the patient as a person. For many doctors this detracts from the satisfaction of the job – especially when they feel that they are being forced to alter their practice on the whim of some misinformed government directive.

As Widgery wrote (and now it might be correct to attribute the adjective 'prophetically') in 1991, 'It is a process of decivilisation in which what doctors prided as a personal relationship between themselves and the patient, is now reshaped by the commodity process. Prevention for populations, service according to need, the family doctors' very idea of themselves as people who had time to grieve with their patients, to share the joy of childbirth, the crisis of illness and the time of day in the corner shop, are swept away.'[148]

Widgery should encourage future generations to make general practice a positive choice. One of the commonest student complaints is that general practice is not scientific enough. It is social work.* This view is

_____

* For example, as one letter in *Student BMJ* stated (in relation to low interest in psychiatry amongst medical students), 'It is my experience that such a lack of interest is not restricted to psychiatry but also applies to care of elderly people and general practice. I wonder if this is because these careers contain the largest element of social work as opposed to straight application of clinical skills and knowledge taught in didactic teaching sessions.'[149]

often countered by pointing out the many ways in which general practice can be science based. GPs can order x-rays, perform electrocardiograms on the premises, do full examinations, etc. Undoubtedly this is true, but David Widgery reminds us of something else. Everyday life (the environment the GP must engage) does not follow Newtonian laws. Social medical work is needed. Social work requires innovative thinking. Social work can inspire.

Widgery demonstrates that GPs are not helpless; they have great political potential at their disposal. The words of MP Dr Howard Stoate articulate this, 'the extraordinary thing about GPs is that they underestimate themselves. They think they are powerless but they are actually not. GPs see two-thirds of a million people every day, far more than consultants do, far more than politicians do, far more than even the clergy. GPs are in a completely unique position. And actually in terms of political hegemony they've actually got by far the most powerful position in society. Because they are professionals, they are looked up to, they are educated, they are generally a fairly switched-on sort of group.'

David Widgery was a remarkable person – someone who tried to achieve the impossible. By doing this he inspired people and it is hoped that he will inspire more. Medicine needs people like him. Society requires people like him. We do not always agree with their views. We may not always approve of their actions, but they are there to ask us what we think – to encourage us to articulate what we believe in.

Think back to the beginning. You were encouraged to think of *Treasure Island* as a parallel to David Widgery's life. There were pirates, fights, bottles of rum and adventures along the way. Whatever happened to the treasure? Talk was of a magnificent wealth – one that promised to save the NHS, stamp out racism and make the world a better place. Did Widgery find this wonderful treasure? If so where is it buried?

Mystery and intrigue remain. If you venture down to the old East End Docks, when the water is still and the moon bright, you may hear people whispering. Some will say Widgery came closer than most; by looking at his life we find the impression of a map. Others are not so sure. They will tell you, 'Widgery sailed in different waters, searching for different treasure. Is the map applicable today? Indeed, how do we know his is *the* map?'.

Widgery left us with only a fragment. Adventurers and treasure seekers should correlate this information with their own charts, interests and hunches – not forgetting the latest weather conditions. Generations will come and go, but the quest will remain. Medicine, idealism and happiness are not fool's gold. They are extremely real and, to those who cherish them, priceless.

References

1 Le Fanu J (1999) *The Rise and Fall of Modern Medicine*. Abacus, London: xviii.
2 www.independent.co.uk.
3 Pendleton D and King J (2002) Values and leadership. *BMJ*. **325**: 1352–5.
4 Shooter M (2002) Students are so full of lists they have forgotten how to listen. *BMJ* **325**: 677.
5 Widgery D (1988) *The National Health*. Hogarth Press, London.
6 Rosen M (1992) David Widgery 1947–92, writer, journalist, doctor and activist – an obituary by Michael Rosen. *The Independent*, 30 October; also www.johng.dial.pipex.com/widgery
7 Fountain N (1992) East side story. Obituary. David Widgery. *The Guardian*, 29 October: 16.
8 Haines A, Heath I and Smith R (2000) Joining together to combat poverty. *BMJ*. **320**: 1.
9 Berger J (1967) *A Fortunate Man: story of country doctor*. Penguin, London.
10 Duncan R (1971) *Selected Writings of Mahatma Gandhi*. Fontana, London: p. 9.
11 Green R (1996) Islington Sixth Form Centre opening evening.
12 Feynman R (1999) *The Pleasure of Finding Things: the best short works of Richard Feynman*. Penguin, London: 182–5.
13 Widgery D (1991) *Some Lives! A GP's East End*. Sinclair and Stevenson, London.
14 Rosen M (2000) Personal interview, 26 March.
15 Gould T (1995) *A Summer Plague: polio and its survivors*. New Haven, London: 229.
16 Ibid: 254.
17 Ibid: 255.
18 Ash J (2000) Personal interview.
19 Phillips D (2002) Personal interview.
20 Fountain N (2002) Personal interview.
21 Ali T (1978) *1968 and After: inside the revolution*. Blond and Briggs, London: vii.
22 Renton D (2002) The life and politics of David Widgery. *Left History* **8/1**: 7–31.
23 Fountain N (2002) Personal interview.
24 Rowbotham S (1997) *A Century of Women: the history of women in Britain and the United States*. Viking, London: 366.
25 Widgery D (1997) Underground press in perspective. *Time Out*; republished in D Widgery (1989) *Preserving Disorder – selected essays 1968–88*: 198.

26 Ibid: 196.
27 Gregory R (2002) Personal interview.
28 Muldoon R (2003) Personal interview.
29 Renton D (2002) The life and politics of David Widgery. From a book review of R Neville (1970) *Playpower*. *Left History* **8/1**: 11.
30 Ibid: 26.
31 Rowbotham S (2002) Personal interview.
32 Widgery D. *Doctor Show – a radical Christmas show*. Widgery archive of writings and videos held by J Ash.
33 Widgery D (1991) *Some Lives! A GP's East End*. Sinclair and Stevenson, London: 4.
34 Ibid: 7.
35 Boomla K (2000) Personal interview, 21 March.
36 Widgery D (1986) *Beating Time; riot 'n' race 'n' rock 'n' roll*. Chatto and Windus, London: 53.
37 Widgery D (1970) Interviewing Johnny Rotten. *Temporary Hoarding*. **14**; also ibid.
38 Renton D (2002) The life and politics of David Widgery. *Left History* **8/1**: 15.
39 Saunders R and Huddle R (1976) Letter. *New Musical Express; Melody Maker; Sounds; Social Worker*; also ibid: 16.
40 Saunders R (2002) Personal interview.
41 Widgery D (1986) B*eating Time; riot 'n' race 'n'rock 'n' roll*. Chatto and Windus, London: 94.
42 Renton D (2002) The life and politics of David Widgery. *Left History* **8/1**: 17.
43 Ibid: 25.
44 Widgery D (1979) Underground press in perspective. *Time Out* [vol: pp]; also D Widgery (1989) *Preserving Disorder – selected essays 1968–88*: 172–3.
45 Ibid: 170.
46 Muldoon R (2002) Personal interview.
47 Widgery D (1987) *Enter Stage Left, New Society*. Also D Widgery (1989) *Preserving Disorder – selected essays 1968–88:* 205.
48 D Widgery (1989) *Meeting Molly. Preserving Disorder – selected essays 1968–88*: 185.
49 Widgery D (1992). In: M Karlin (1989, repeated 1992 Channel 4) *Utopias*.
50 Berger J (1967) *A Fortunate Man: story of country doctor*. Penguin, London: 79.
51 Emerson RW.   http://www.brainyquote.com/quotes/authors/r/ralph_waldo_emerson.html
52 Smith R (2001) Why are doctors so unhappy? *BMJ*. **322**: 1073–4.
53 Jakeman N (2001) It's not all doom and gloom. Letters, *BMJ*. **322**: 1361.
54 BMJ Survey (2001) *Why Are Doctors So Unhappy?* 4–17 May. http://bmj.com/cgi/content/full/322/7294/DC4
55 Dostoevsky F (1866) *Crime and Punishment*. Wordsworth Editions Ltd, London: 334.
56 Porter R (1999) *The Greatest Benefit to Mankind: a medical history of humanity*. Fontana Press, London.
57 Black, Sir D (chairman) (1980) *Inequalities in Health*. Department of Health and Social Security, London.

58 Tucker A (2002) Sir Douglas Black obituary. *The Guardian*, 14 September.

59 Rivett G (1997) *From Cradle to Grave. Fifty years of the NHS*. King's Fund Publishing, London: 298.

60 Webster C (1988) The Health Service Since the War. HMSO, London: 137.

61 Shaw M, Dorling D, Gordon D and Davey Smith D (1999) *The Widening Gap: health inequalities*. Policy Press, Bristol; 169.

62 Widgery D (1989) *Preserving Disorder – selected essays 1968–88*. Pluto Press, London: 189.

63 Fitzpatrick M (2000) *The Tyranny of Health: doctors and the regulation of lifestyle*. Routledge, London: 162.

64 Stewart J (1999) '*The Battle for Health': a political history of the Socialist Medical Association, 1930–51* (History of Medicine in Context). Ashgate Publishing, Aldershot: 103.

65 Navarro V (1978) *Class Struggle, the State and Medicine: an historical and contemporary analysis of the medical sector in Great Britain* (Medicine in Society). Robertson, London.

66 Widgery D (1979) I'm not going to work on Maggie's farm. *Socialist Worker*. Also D Widgery (1989) *Preserving Disorder – selected essays 1968–88*: 172.

67 Widgery D (1976) *The Left in Britain 1956–68*. Penguin, Middlesex; also D Widgery (1989) *Preserving Disorder – selected essays 1968–88*. Pluto Press, London: xiii.

68 Widgery D (1988) *The National Health*. Hogarth Press, London: xv–xvi.

69 Rivett G (1997) *From Cradle to Grave. Fifty years of the NHS*. King's Fund Publishing, London: 412.

70 Widgery D (1974) Death of a hospital. *Socialist Worker*. Also D Widgery (1989) *Preserving Disorder – selected essays 1968–88*: 141.

71 Rivett G (1997) *From Cradle to Grave. Fifty years of the NHS*. King's Fund Publishing, London: 277.

72 Widgery D (1988) *The National Health*. Hogarth Press, London: 161.

73 Ibid: 166.

74 Ibid: 159.

75 Ibid: 162.

76 Ibid: 169.

77 Ibid: 170.

78 Widgery D (1974) Death of a hospital. _*Socialist Worker*. Also D Widgery (1989) *Preserving Disorder – selected essays 1968–88*: 142.

79 Berdoe E (1883) www.members.aol.com/_ht_a/dbryantmd/home.html

80 Ober W (1973) Chekhov amongst the doctors. In: *Essays on the History of Medicine*. Selected from the Bulletin of the New York Academy of Medicine, Science History Publications (1976) The History of Medicine Series no. 47. 209–23.

81 MacDonald R (2002) Commentary: are content good doctors good doctors? *BMJ*. **325**: 686.

82 Russell B (1935) *In Praise of Idleness*. (1967) Unwin Books, London: 14.

83 Ibid: 21.

84 Salinsky J (2001) *Medicine and Literature: the doctor's companion to the classics*. Radcliffe Medical Press, Oxford: 2.

85   Coope R (1952) *The Quiet Art, A Doctor's Anthology*. E&S Livingstone, Edinburgh and London.

86   Gould T (1995) *A Summer Plague: polio and its survivors*. New Haven, London: 254.

87   Ali T (1978) *1968 and After: inside the revolution*. Blond and Briggs, London.

88   Widgery D (1992) *Blueprint*. Widgery archive of writings and videos held by J Ash.

89   Widgery D (1989) *Preserving Disorder – selected essays 1968–88*. Pluto Press, London: 154.

90   Renton D (2004) David Widgery: The Poetics of Propaganda. In: D Renton. *Dissident Marxism* 2e, London: 205–34.

91   Renton D (2002) The life and politics of David Widgery. *Left History* **8/1**: 27.

92   Ash J (2000) Personal interview.

93   Rivett G (1997) *From Cradle to Grave. Fifty years of the NHS*. King's Fund Publishing, London: 357.

94   Widgery D (1988) *The National Health*. Hogarth Press, London: 1.

95   Widgery D (1989) *Preserving Disorder – selected essays 1968–88*. Pluto Press, London: 95.

96   Widgery D (1988) *The National Health*. Hogarth Press, London: 45.

97   Ibid: 46.

98   Ibid: 51.

99   Ibid: 52.

100   Ibid: xvi.

101   Widgery D (1989) The National Health: A radical perspective. The Hogarth Press, London: 149.

102   Widgery D (1989) *Preserving Disorder – selected essays 1968–88*. Pluto Press, London: 190.

103   (1988) Review of *The National Health*. CHIC, October.

104   Smith R (1988) Review of *The National Health*. *Observer*, 3 July.

105   Hoggart L (1988) The Tory Shame. *Socialist Worker Review*, October.

106   Robinson J (1989) Book Reviews. *Journal of Advanced Nursing* **4**: 6.

107   Widgery D (1988) *The National Health*. Hogarth Press, London: 170.

108   Widgery D (1986) *Beating Time; riot 'n' race 'n' rock 'n' roll*. Chatto and Windus, London: 36.

109   Bosley M (1989) *7 Days. Health Service Leads*, 17 June.

110   Widgery D (1991) *Some Lives! A GP's East End*. Sinclair and Stevenson, London: 7.

111   Ibid: 44.

112   Ibid: 47.

113   Ibid: 60.

114   Ibid: 198.

115   Ibid: 188.

116   Ibid: 21–4.

117   Ibid: 121.

118   Ibid: 75–6.

119   Ibid: 4.

120 Harman H (1991) East Side Story. *Independent on Sunday*, 28 July.
121 Iliffe S (1991) Review of *Some Lives! BMJ.* **303**: 256.
122 (1992) GP can say 'I told you so' after Canary Wharf fails. *GP News.*
123 Widgery D (1968) Over and under. *Oz* **17**.
124 Smith R (2003) Personal interview.
125 Heath I (2000) Personal interview.
126 Widgery D (1990) Gone West? *BMJ.* **300**: 1279.
127 Myers D (1992) Letter. *BMJ.* **304**: 576.
128 Widgery D (1991) The prince and the psychiatrists. *BMJ.* **303**: 723.
129 Tudor Hart J (1988) *A New Kind of Doctor.* Merlin Press, London: 2.
130 Turner T (2003) Personal interview.
131 Widgery D (1976) *The Left in Britain 1956–68.* Penguin, Middlesex: 437.
132 Heath I (1995) *The Mystery of General Practice.* The Nuffield Provincial Hospitals Trust, London.
133 Warden J (1997) Focus: Westminster – New Doctors in the House. *BMJ.* **314**: 1781.
134 Widgery D (1970) *International Socialism.* Also D Widgery (1989) *Preserving Disorder – selected essays 1968–88*: 89.
135 Bethel A (1992) *Limehouse Doctor.* Produced by Double Exposure.
136 Staff writer (1991) *GP Magazine* Cutting in Juliet Ash's archive.
137 Widgery D (1983) Doctoring. *New Internationalist* Also D Widgery (1989) *Preserving Disorder – selected essays 1968–88*: 188.
138 Balint M (1957) *The Doctor, His Patient and the Illness.* Pitman Medical, London.
139 Widgery D (1988) Too much monkey business. *New Society*, February; also D Widgery (1989) *Preserving Disorder – selected essays 1968–88*: 209.
140 Gould T (1995) *A Summer Plague: polio and its survivors.* New Haven, London: 256.
141 Renton D (2002) The life and politics of David Widgery. *Left History* **8/1**: 22.
142 Greenhalgh T (1993) One hell of a doctor. *BMJ.* **306**: 1009.
143 Bloch M (1954) *The Historian's Craft.* Manchester University Press, Manchester.
144 Tudor Hart J (1988) A New Kind of Doctor. Merlin Press, London: 332.
145 NHS Confederation (2002) The problem with unhappy doctors – what are the causes and what can we do? NHS Confederation, London: 4.
146 Ibid: 9.
147 Willis J (2001) *Friends in Low Places.* Radcliffe Medical Press, Oxford: 90.
148 Widgery D (1991) GP mourns the dying East End. *GP Magazine*, July: 32.
149 Oates T (2003) Letter. *Student BMJ*, July.

Index

Locators in italics refer to photographs. DW to David Widgery.